# Taking the Vegan Challenge

A Guide to Going Vegan
to Lose up to 20 Pounds in 30 Days

**Vegan Diet for Beginners**

*Based on Scientific Research*

A.I. Jäger

All rights reserved. No part of this book may be reproduced or transmitted in any form or by any means without written permission from the author.

This book is intended as a reference volume only, not as a medical manual. Nothing written in this book should be viewed as a substitute for competent medical care. The information given here is designed to help you make more informed decisions about your health.
It is not intended as a substitute for any treatment that may have been prescribed by your doctor. If you suspect that you have a medical problem, we urge you to seek competent medical help.

Copyright © Anna I. Jaeger

All rights reserved.
First Edition February, 2015

ISBN-13: 978-1507711262
ISBN-10: 1507711263

# Content

Introduction ..................................................................................... 7
1| Being Vegan .................................................................................. 8
2| The Benefits of Going Vegan................................................... 11
3| Debunking the Myths of Veganism ...................................... 14
4| Going Vegan – Tips and Tricks for Getting Started ....... 22
    *The Do's and Don'ts of Your New Diet*................................ *23*
5| The 30 Day Vegan Challenge ................................................ 28
    *Additional money saving tips for vegan grocery shopping* ............. *31*
6| Conclusion...................................................................................34
7| More Groundbreaking Studies ..............................................35
8| Bonus-Chapter: 7-Day Mealplan Recipes ........................36
Monday.............................................................................................37
    *Breakfast: Blueberry Pancakes* ................................................. *37*
    *Snack: Vanilla Chia Pudding* .....................................................*39*
    *Lunch: Pesto Pasta* ........................................................................ *41*
    *Dinner: Black Bean Wrap*............................................................*43*
Tuesday.............................................................................................45
    *Breakfast: French Toast*............................................................. *45*
    *Snack: Banana Blueberry Bars* ................................................ *47*
    *Lunch: Kale, Lemon & Cilantro Sandwich* ........................... *49*
    *Dinner: Quinoa Teriyaki* ..............................................................*51*
Wednesday .....................................................................................53
    *Breakfast: Cinnamon Berry Oatmeal* ..................................... *53*
    *Snack: Watermelon Salad*........................................................... *55*
    *Lunch: Black Bean Tacos* ............................................................ *57*
    *Dinner: Shepard's Pie*....................................................................*59*

## Thursday .................................................. 61
### Breakfast: Spicy Southern Grits .................................................. 61
### Snack: Peanut Butter and Jelly Smoothie .................................................. 63
### Lunch: Black Beans and Rice .................................................. 65
### Dinner: Vegetable Pasta .................................................. 67

## Friday .................................................. 69
### Breakfast: Blueberry Muffins .................................................. 69
### Snack: Apple Cookies (A healthier cookie option) .................................................. 71
### Lunch: Mac n' Cheese .................................................. 73
### Dinner: Chickpea Chili .................................................. 75

## Saturday .................................................. 77
### Breakfast: Breakfast Cookies .................................................. 77
### Snack: Strawberry Banana Popsicles .................................................. 79
### Lunch: Black Bean Veggie Burger .................................................. 81
### Dinner: Lasagna Rolls .................................................. 84

## Sunday .................................................. 86
### Breakfast: Breakfast Tortillas .................................................. 86
### Snack: Baked Sweet Potato Chips .................................................. 88
### Lunch: Tomato Soup .................................................. 90
### Dinner: Tortilla Casserole .................................................. 92

## Dessert – Healthier Options .................................................. 94
### Peach Cobbler .................................................. 94
### Raw Apple Crumble .................................................. 96
### Dark Chocolate Brownies .................................................. 98
### Piña Colada Smoothie .................................................. 100
### Chocolate Mousse .................................................. 102
### Banana Cream Pie .................................................. 104
### Apple Strudel .................................................. 106

## NEW – Available Now .................................................. 108

## Recommendations .................................................. 109

## Disclaimer & Legal Information .................................................. 110

# Introduction

If you are reading this book, you are about to embark on a journey that will change your life. You have probably already read something about the vegan diet and what it can do for you but the internet is loaded with myths, half-truths, and bias criticisms so it's hard to separate fact from fiction. This comes from both sides. For every omnivore out there criticizing the vegan diet as unhealthy or boring; there's a vegan making wild and unproven claims about what it means to be vegan.

With this book, you can take a breath and finally learn what's true, what's false, and what you need to do become vegan and live the healthy, happy life you've always dreamed of living. In these short chapters, many of your questions about the vegan diet will be answered. You may have stumbled upon this diet in hopes of losing weight. On that count, you will not be disappointed. When done right, the vegan diet can help you lose all those unwanted pounds quickly and safely. And this book will help you do it right!

- As you read through these chapters, you'll learn
- what exactly it means to be vegan
- some of the amazing benefits you'll get if you go vegan
- the facts behind 10 of the most common myths about the vegan diet
- simple and effective tips and tricks for starting your vegan diet and sticking to it, and;
- a complete diet and budget plan for a 30 day vegan challenge that will help you lose weight, improve your health, and feel better (all or just $35 per week)!

Say goodbye to those unhealthy and untested crash diets and fad diets and say hello to the scientifically proven, healthy, and effective vegan diet.

Keep on reading and get ready to make a change in your life that will actually make a difference!

# 1|
# Being Vegan

There are a lot of different ideas about what it actually means to be vegan. There are even different "levels" of being vegan. So it's understandably a little confusing to hear about the vegan diet and figure out what people are actually talking about when they use the word. The great thing is that our bodies are capable of absorbing nutrients from a staggering variety of foods. But the first thing you need to know is that people are primarily herbivores. According to biologists and anthropologists, humans are herbivores who are not well suited to eating meat.

Today, many people have made the assumption that we need to eat tons of meat to survive. But this is not true. We are not carnivores. We lack both the physical characteristics of carnivores and the instinct that drives us to kill animals and devour their raw carcasses. Read author John Robbins' discussion of the anatomical differences between humans and carnivores to learn more.

In fact, many of our ancestors didn't eat very much meat. Hunting an animal was dangerous and hard work so our ancestors did it rarely. Before we invented tools, hunting wasn't done at all. The only meat that our ancestors at this time was whatever they could pick off the carcass of an animal that something else killed. Usually, there wasn't much left but bones and few tough bits of flesh. So for millions of years, humans ate meat very rarely.

That is what our digestive tracts adapted to deal with: primarily plant based diets with the occasional piece of meat. This is why a piece of meat will sit in your intestines for a lot longer than a piece of vegetable. In some cases, meat can actually start to rot before your body has managed to fully digest it. This can cause a lot of health problems which is why the meat heavy diet that many people in the United States and Europe eat is associated with poor health.

The moral of the story is: just because we can eat meat doesn't mean we should be eating it with every single meal of every single day. This is like saying that because we can digest some alcohol without dying means that we should drink a bottle of vodka with every meal. If you are going to eat meat, you need to give your body time to properly digest it and you need to make sure that you are getting enough plant foods that are high in fiber to help it along.

The next thing you need to know is that being vegan is not the same as vegetarian. Vegetarians simply cut meat out of their diet. In some cases, they will even continue to eat fish. Becoming vegetarian can be a great first step into the diet since you can get used to cutting out meat before you go the rest of the way to become a full vegan.

The simplest definition of "vegan" would be someone who does not eat any food that comes from animals: meat, fish, dairy, eggs, gelatin, and so on. This is sometimes called "dietary vegan" because these people only practice veganism in relation to what they eat. Some go even further and don't use any products made from animals like leather, suede, wool or certain dyes. Still others go further and include insect products on that list like honey or silk. These last two are usually known as "ethical vegans" because they are trying to cut every single animal or insect based product from their lives and usually do so based on ethical reasons.

To go this far and avoid every possible animal product takes a lot of care and planning because there are many things that you wouldn't immediately realize contain animal products in them even though they do. So, while it is a valiant effort, it's also a never ending journey to constantly check the products you are using and make sure they are totally vegan in this sense of the word.

There is another unofficial category of vegan called "junk vegan." This refers to those people who cut all animal products out of their diet but do not take care to eat a healthy, balanced variety of foods. Instead, they eat mainly vegan-friendly junk food. This kind of diet leads to a lot of health problems and can actually cause weight gain instead of weight loss (just as junk food always tends to cause weight gain even in omnivores).

For this book, we are concerned with the vegan diet so we won't go into throwing out all your leather shoes and wool coats. If you are considering the vegan diet for ethical reasons then taking that extra step is something you will want to look into on your own.

If you do want to cut out insect products (like honey) out as well, you can find other substitutes. There is a natural sweetener made from the plant stevia that will also work but, depending on where you live, it might not be as easy to come by as honey.

As you can see, vegan can mean many different things for different people. What it means for you will depend on what your reasons for adopting the diet are. If you are like many people who hope to use the vegan diet to lose weight and get healthier, then cutting out non-food products made from animals or insect products is unnecessary. If, on the other hand, you are concerned about the wellbeing of animals or environmental sustainability, then you may want to adopt a more strict definition of vegan.

This book will give you a thorough introduction of the vegan diet in the least strict sense: just cutting out meat, fish, and animal food products (dairy, eggs, gelatin, etc). You can do additional research if you want to learn more about how to cut out other animal products.

# 2|
# The Benefits of Going Vegan

Many critics will tell you that being vegan is unhealthy and has no benefits. We'll deal with these criticisms in the next chapter where we work through the 10 most common myths and why they are false. But first, let's talk about the benefits that going vegan does have.

There are actually quite a few benefits if you plan your diet well to include all the nutritious whole plant foods that you need so it would be impossible for this chapter to include all of them. Instead, we'll just talk about a few of the biggest benefits.

- **Weight Loss**

One of the main reasons many people even start the vegan diet is to lose weight. Because the diet is naturally low in saturated fats, trans fats, and refined sugar, people lose weight surprisingly fast. The diet is also high in complex carbohydrates which are high in fiber and often also protein (while also being low in calories). This means you will naturally eat less and feel full for much longer after the meal so you'll be losing weight without having to starve yourself.

- **Improved Health**

For many of the same reasons that it helps you lose weight, the vegan diet is also great for your health. By eating a diet full of fruits, vegetables, legumes, and other nutritious plant foods; you'll be getting a full range of nutrients without any of the harmful additives or fats that are often a part of the average meat eater's diet. Most people tend to neglect plant foods even though these are essential sources of vitamins and minerals that you simply can't find in meat. Migraine or headache sufferers who go on vegan diets frequently discover relief from their migraines. Reduction in dairy, meat, and eggs is often tied to alleviation of allergy symptoms.

Many vegans report much fewer runny noses and congestion problems. Eating a healthy vegan diet has also shown to prevent a number of diseases (cardiovascular disease, high cholesterol, high blood pressure, macular degeneration, fungus, cataracts, acid reflux disease, arthritis, osteoporosis, eczema, chronic fatigue syndrome, asthma). Your weight will go down, your skin will turn into beautiful, clear, healthy-looking skin (some people call it „Glow"), your whole body will be working more efficiently, and you'll just feel better overall.

- **Improved Taste**

By eliminating meat and animal products from your diet, you'll open yourself up to the many possibilities of the plant based diet. Even if you've never thought of yourself as much of a chef or even a foodie; the vegan diet will have you experimenting with all kinds of flavor combinations and developing a newfound talent for creating exciting new dishes using nothing but nutritious and flavorful fruits, vegetables, and other plant foods.

- **Stronger Nails and Healthier Hair**

Healthy vegan diets are also responsible for much stronger, healthier nails. Nail health is said to be an indicator of overall health. Many who follow vegan diets report that their hair becomes stronger, has more body, and looks shinier and healthier.

- **Better Sleep**

A study on the physiological benefits of a vegan diet found that subjects who switched to eating purely plant-based reported an improvement in the quality of their sleep. Many vegans report to sleeping for less time each night but waking up more refreshed.

- **Reduced Body Odor**

Eliminating dairy and red meat from the diet significantly reduces body odor. Going vegan means smelling better. Vegans frequently experience a reduction in bad breath, as well. Imagine waking up in the morning and not having morning breath.

- **Improved Cooking Skills**

Just as your ability to recognize and combine flavors creatively will improve, so too will your ability to use more and more complex techniques in the kitchen. Even if your current cooking skills are limited to boiling a pot of water; you'll soon find yourself roasting, sautéing, searing, and baking with the best of them. The vegan diet will allow you to unleash your inner chef so that you can eat a delicious variety of different kinds of meals.

- **Increased Self Confidence**

As you start to look and feel better, your confidence will also start to increase. You'll feel comfortable in your own skin and you'll feel proud to go out and show the world the new you. You'll also be able to take pride in your new found skills in the kitchen and the fact that you finally took charge and took control of your life by changing your diet, losing weight, and getting healthy.

- **Better Mood and More Energy**

A better, more nutritious diet doesn't just mean better physical health; it also means better psychological health. A balanced diet will help stabilize your hormones which will stabilize your mood, making you a happier, less stressed person overall. You'll also have more energy because the fiber and protein rich carbohydrates you are eating will stabilize your blood glucose levels so that you have sustained energy throughout the day rather than dealing with the peaks and crashes of energy that often come with the average meat eater's diet.

Overall, you will be able to lose those stubborn unwanted pounds while transforming yourself into the happier, healthier you that you were always meant to be. If you're still not sure going vegan is the right thing for you, read on to the next chapter to learn the true facts about veganism that finally put the myths to rest once and for all.

# 3 |
# Debunking the Myths of Veganism

In the ongoing debates about what is and is not healthy, myths abound on both sides. The fact of the matter is there is more than one way to be healthy. Likewise, there is more than one way to be unhealthy. There are a lot of unhealthy foods out there and there are also a lot of foods that become unhealthy if you eat too much of them.

The key to being healthy is eating a wide variety of foods to make sure you've got all your bases covered. Even if you cut out all animal products, you can still get enough variety. If you've been considering a vegan diet but are worried because you've heard a lot of stories about vitamin deficiencies and other health problems, this chapter should help put you at ease. Here, we will go over 10 of the most common myths you have probably heard about vegans and a thorough explanation about why they aren't true (or, at least, don't have to be true if you are smart about it).

**Myth: Vegans Don't Get Enough Protein**

Calorie for calorie, yes, animal foods have more protein. But that does not mean protein is only found in animals. Many plant foods are loaded with protein and it's actually extremely easy to get your full daily requirement of protein without eating a single animal product. Grains, legumes, beans, nuts, and seeds are all tiny protein powerhouses.

You may have also heard the counterargument that there might be protein in plant foods but they don't have "complete" proteins. This argument is based on the idea that protein is not just one component of food but a combination of 9 essential amino acids. In animal products, these 9 amino acids are already combined into "complete" proteins. The myth is that there are no plant foods that contain all 9 amino acids.

The fact is almost every single edible thing on the planet contains some amount of all the amino acids. This includes many plant foods that contain great levels of all 9 of the essential amino acids (pumpkin seeds, black beans, quinoa, and soy just to name a few).

There are also many plant foods that contain high levels of certain essential amino acids that can be paired with other plant foods that are high in the missing ones. This art of protein combining is something every health conscious vegan has mastered. In fact, protein combining has been going on long before we were aware that protein (or any other nutrient) existed.

Beans and rice (a staple of Mexican cuisine) or soybeans and rice (a Japanese staple) are excellent examples of two foods that combine to make a complete protein. Beans and soybeans are exceptionally high in the exact amino acids that rice is exceptionally low in (and vice versa) so that when put together, you are getting a meal with all 9 amino acids represented.

The bottom line is it's just as easy to get enough protein with a vegan diet as it is with any other diet (except, I guess, a protein-free diet if that exists).

### Myth: The Vegan Diet Is Too Expensive

One of the first things people associate with the vegan diet (after "a whole lot of vegetables") is money. It seems that eating so much fresh produce and fancy foods is expensive. And, sure, you can spend quite a lot of money on food if you are a vegan. But you can also spend a lot of money on food even if you are not a vegan.

Meat is usually more expensive pound for pound than any vegetable you'll see at the store. The only reason you might see a spike in your grocery bill is if your switching from a diet of cheap, processed foods to a diet of healthy, fresh plant foods.

Processed foods are full of preservatives and chemicals that keep them from spoiling meaning the stores can keep them on the shelf for longer which cuts costs on their end and allows them to mark down the price. In the end, though, you might save a few bucks but you are also eating those preservatives and chemicals which your body doesn't know how to handle. They end up either poisoning you or, in the absolute best case scenario, getting stored as fat until your body can figure out what else to do with it.

These same foods may be cheaper than fresh produce but they also aren't as satisfying. You inflate from all the extra stored fat but you don't feel full for very long because there actually wasn't much nutrition in it. In order to get that full feeling you're looking, you need to eat foods that have something to offer. Fresh, unprocessed plant foods are packed with nutrients which means you end up needing way less of them to feel full (and that full feeling will last for much, much longer).

If the price tag on healthy plant foods still scares you, continue reading to chapter 5 where you'll learn how to eat a completely healthy, unprocessed vegan diet for just $35 per week (per person). You'll spend less, eat better, and eat less because you'll feel more satisfied from each meal.

## Myth: You Will Get a Vitamin B12 Deficiency if You Go Vegan

This is one of the trickier myths. It is true that vitamin B12 is not found naturally in any plants. This is because plants don't make it and don't use it so they have no method of storing of it. It is also true that a vitamin B12 deficiency will cause serious health problems. With that said, there are simple and affordable ways to get around this as a vegan.

Today, there are many foods that have been fortified with vitamin B12 in a totally vegan way. They use a complex combination of bacteria which when put all in one place, work together to produce the vitamin. This product is then injected into various foods or even right into fresh produce which is capable of absorbing it. So if you check for B12 fortified foods, you can make sure your diet is getting enough in this way.

Any easier (and cheaper) way to do it, however, is to take a supplement. Look for vegan B12 supplements. There are a few different products out there but what you want is preferably a "sublingual" supplement with either 25 micrograms per day or 2,500 micrograms per week. Sublingual just means you stick under your tongue and it dissolves.

Your body absorbs it more easily in this form. You will see a lot of 2,500 microgram supplements in bottles that recommend taking them for daily use. But this is just an attempt to get you to spend more money. At that dosage, you can just take one per week and get your full weekly requirement. A bottle of 90 tablets (2,500 micrograms each) will run you about $10 to $15. This is extremely cheap when you consider that 90 tablets will last you 90 weeks (or nearly 2 years) meaning you would spend $0.11 to $0.16 per week to meet your full vitamin B12 requirements. Plus, taking one tablet per week is easy and if you eat a well balanced diet (and get enough sunlight), this is the only supplement you'll need to take!

## Myth: Plant Foods Don't Have Enough Calcium, Iron, Vitamin D, or Zinc

One hobby that critics really seem to enjoy is making the claim that plant foods somehow are vitamin deficient. This is in spite of the decades of research which show all the different kinds of vitamins and minerals that are found in plants (and the fact that attempting to eat an all meat diet would leave you with more deficiencies than you could count).

In addition to protein and B12, critics claim that plant foods don't contain enough calcium, iron, zinc, or vitamin D. In the first three cases, this is absolutely not true. There are many plant based sources of all of these things and if you follow the diet plan from chapter 5, you'll get plenty of all three of them. When it comes to vitamin D, not even most animal foods (except for certain species of fish) contain it naturally.

Vitamin D is only found naturally in a few select foods. In most cases, if you see vitamin D on the label, it's because it was added in later. You can easily find vegan foods that have also been fortified with vitamin D. You could also eat shitake mushrooms which are one of the few foods that naturally contain some vitamin D (although you'll need to eat a lot because they don't have much so it would be as pricey as it is yummy).

The good news is that if you live somewhere where the sun shines which is literally everywhere unless you are living in the depths of the ocean or confine yourself to a cave all year round (in which case, how are you reading this ebook?) then you can get your full daily requirement of vitamin D just by sitting outside and soaking up some sun rays for about 15 minutes. A couple notes on using the sun for vitamin D: it needs to be direct sunlight (not through a window or a cloud or a layer of sunscreen lotion) and you need to be careful if you burn easily. For most sunburn-prone people, 15 minutes is just short enough to get your vitamin D without getting burned.

After that 15 minutes, though, put on some sunscreen. Another thing to consider: if you live somewhere with these pesky things called seasons, especially winter, you may need to take a vitamin D supplement or increase the amount of vitamin D fortified foods in your diet during the dark winter months.

## Myth: Omega 3 Fatty Acids Are Only in Animal Foods

First of all, what on earth are omega 3 fatty acids and why are we suddenly caring about them? The simple answer: they are type of unsaturated fat that has been shown to be essential for heart health, brain health, and overall cardiovascular health. Basically, it's lubricating your whole system and keeping things running smoothly. It cleans the plaque buildup in your veins and does all sorts of other neat things you can read more about if it interests you.

Second of all, it is found in a lot of foods aside from animal products. In fact, it is found in most natural foods. **There are plenty of plant sources that contain the right balance of omega 3 to omega 6 and can provide you with more than enough to meet your needs.**

The recommended daily intake of omega 3 fatty acids is 1,200 milligrams. This is just an estimate, though, because the amount you need daily depends on how much omega 6 you are eating. You should try to get them to be at least equal with each other. So if you eat 1,200 milligrams of omega 3; then you need to limit your omega 6 to 1,200 milligrams as well.

The best way to do this is to eat seeds. Flax seeds are the best option. In just one ounce of flax seeds, you get 6,388 milligrams of omega 3 (and only 1,655 milligrams of omega 6). So this single ounce will help offset any of the other omega 6 rich foods you might be eating (like certain oils and nuts).

Aside from flax seeds, there's also chia seeds and hemp seeds. Admittedly, these guys can get pretty expensive (especially if you're eating an ounce a day). Alternatives are to buy ground flaxseed meal and get creative with the oven (it's usually around $5 or $6 for 2 pounds of meal).

### Myth: You Can't Build Muscle without Meat

Fact: muscles are made up of protein which is made up of 9 amino acids which, as we have already discussed, are all bountiful in plant foods. So if you want to be a big, beefy bodybuilder, going vegan will not stop you. You can get as much protein (and as much complete protein) as your heart desires from a completely plant based diet.

In fact, you can get all that protein without taking all the saturated fats and LDL (bad) cholesterol that comes with it. If you need to eat a protein heavy diet, it is actually recommended to get most of that protein from plant sources because if you eat as much meat as you would need to meet your requirements, you'll also be increasing your risk for heart problems, dangerously high blood pressure, crazy high LDL cholesterol, and constipation to boot.

Loading up on quinoa and lentils will do your body much better than eating a giant hunk of steak for every meal of the day. Not to mention, it takes your body a lot longer to break down and absorb the nutrients from meat than it does from plant foods. So, even if becoming a bodybuilder is not your goal, you're more than capable of getting the nutrients you need to stay healthy and strong from a vegan diet. Muscles require protein and exercise. The vegan diet has the protein covered so if you want to build muscle, all you have to do is start hitting the gym.

### Myth: Vegans Are Always Hungry

This is a weird myth but, unfortunately, quite wide spread. People seem to think that meat is the only thing that makes you feel full. In reality, your body feels full whenever your stomach has food to digest in it. As soon as it's finished breaking it down and sent it on to your intestines, you feel hungry again. If you eat foods that digest easily (like simple carbohydrates or liquid based foods), you'll feel hungry again sooner because your stomach will finish its work quickly.

So, if you want to feel full for longer and keep your appetite under control, eat foods that keep your stomach busy: protein and complex carbohydrates. As you have read twice already, plant foods contain plenty of protein. They also contain a lot of complex carbohydrates (mainly in the form of fiber) which meat contains very little of unless you are in the habit of eating animal hooves.

If you eat a balanced vegan meal high in protein and complex carbohydrates, you will actually stay full for a longer amount of time than your friend who just ate a processed, preservative-soaked fast food burger (and you'll have eaten a fraction of the calories!)

### Myth: The Vegan Diet Causes Chronic Fatigue

Fatigue happens when the glucose levels in your blood are low. This happens when your body has already processed and used all the energy from the food you ate. So, if you do not eat enough or eat foods that digest too quickly, you will experience fatigue whether you are vegan or not.

To avoid fatigue, you need to a diet rich in protein and complex carbohydrates which digest slowly and help maintain stable levels of glucose in your blood. You can easily do this on a vegan diet with the right planning. If you follow the 30 day plan from chapter 5, you'll safely avoid low glucose levels (and, therefore, fatigue).

### Myth: The Vegan Diet Is Bland and Boring

After exhausting all the health related myths about being vegan, critics will often resort to claiming that the vegan diet is just plain boring. In fact, the exact opposite is true. By going vegan, you have to get creative about what you eat. You combine lots of different fruits, vegetables, grains, legumes, beans, and seasonings to create meals that are not only extremely healthy but also amazingly flavorful—a lot more flavorful than just eat a plain steak.

The people who claim that a vegan diet is bland are also usually the same people who eat the same 5 meals week in and week out and don't bother to experiment with new foods and new flavor combinations. Variety is the spice of life. And, as it turns out, spice is also the spice of life. If you do it right, the vegan diet will be a lot more interesting and flavorful than the average person's omnivorous diet.

### Myth: Going Vegan Is Too Hard

It might seem like a completely different kind of lifestyle and, in some ways, it is. If you grew up with animal products included in every meal, you might have a hard time imagining what kinds of meals you'll be eating if there's no meat, cheese, milk, or butter involved. I won't tell you it's an easy change. But I can say with confidence that you will adapt to it quicker than you thought you would and the benefits of doing so will keep you motivated.

Once you really start exploring all of your options with the vegan diet, you'll hardly miss animal products. Most people see going vegan as a limitation since you are cutting out a whole category of food that most people have grown up eating. But it's more like an opportunity to explore foods that you have been neglecting your entire life. It's sort of like when you are child and you pretend the floor is lava so you can't walk on it. You don't do it to limit yourself; you do it so you can have fun exploring new ways of getting around the house (often by jumping around on the furniture until your parents yell at you.) The normal way of doing things might seem like the best but the creative way of doing things is almost always more fun.

Your diet is what you make it. If you buy the same ingredients and make the same dishes, it will get boring whether there are animal products in it or not. On the other hand, if you have fun with cooking, there's really no end to the possibilities.

# 4|
# Going Vegan –
# Tips and Tricks for Getting Started

Before you take the 30 day vegan challenge which you'll read more about in the next chapter, there are few tips and tricks that you should have in mind to make sure that your journey to health, happiness, and weight loss is as successful and rewarding as it should be. In this chapter, you'll read about the do's and don'ts of going vegan.

Unfortunately, a lot of well-intentioned people start the vegan diet without doing their research. They all tend to make the same mistakes since they don't know any better and end up having bad results. A lot of the myths you read about in chapter 3 are based on these unhealthy mistakes that these people have made.

A lot of these mistakes (like loading up on processed, artificial foods rather than fresh, whole foods) are the same kinds of things that non-vegans do as well. In fact, all of the tips and tricks discussed in this chapter are actually things that people on any diet should be following in order to lose weight or otherwise improve their health.

So, even if you choose to give up the vegan diet after you successfully complete the 30 day challenge, you should continue to follow these same tips even when you bring animal products back into the mix. Although, if you do it right, you'll probably find that you are enjoying the benefits and the food varieties of your new vegan diet more than you ever thought possible. Don't be surprised if you find yourself still motivated to be vegan long after these first 30 days are up.

# The Do's and Don'ts of Your New Diet

### 1. Don't Eat Processed or Refined Foods

Processed foods are sneaky devils. They're full of indigestible, nutrition-poor compounds that clog up your body and cause untold amounts of damage to every single system. These are things like cookies (not counting any delicious, homemade vegan ones), TV dinners, pre-made soups, or pretty much anything with a longer life expectancy than you. If there's an ingredient in the list that you can't immediately recognize, skip it. If it's loaded with refined sugar, skip it. If it's got any amount of corn syrup at all, run for your life! As a vegan (or any other kind of human being), you need a diet of whole, unprocessed foods. These are packed with nutrients, more satisfying, and help fight diseases rather than help cause them.

### 2. Eat Starch!

Eating more starches (potatoes, beans, corn) and vegetables is the perfect way to decrease your appetite and increase the nutrients in your diet. Incorporate starches and vegetables into your daily meals as much as possible and it will reduce hunger and help your body feel great. Both raw and cooked vegetables are great choices for your diet and will help you fill up so you are not eating as much sugar and other foods.

Getting rid of all the negative foods which are contributing to your diabetes is easier said than done. Your body has come to depend on these unhealthy foods and will start to withdraw as you take these foods away. It is essential that you are building up your vitamins and minerals with as many healthy vegetables as you can during the process of stopping your unhealthy foods. Keep thinking about how great you are going to feel when you have reversed your diabetes!

As you cut out sugar from your diet in the form of refined carbohydrates, refined sugars and processed foods, your body will feel energetic. Still, it is important to give yourself plenty of extra time to rest and for sleeping. Sleep is a necessary part to your body giving up on the unhealthy foods and you starting to eat more healthy foods.

Think about how all your friends and family will be coming to you for help. How they will look up to you for all the hard work you have done. This is your chance to show everyone you are ready to make a change.

### 3. Do Make Every Meal Colorful

One of the reasons people think going vegan is hard is because you have to worry about getting all the nutrients. Here's a quick wakeup call: everyone has to worry about getting all the nutrients they need (or, at least, they should be). One easy tip for making sure the meal you are eating has a nice balance of all the nutrients you need is to make sure it is colorful. The color of a plant can often work as a hint about what kind of vitamins and minerals are inside it. For example, beta-carotene (part of the vitamin A family) in large quantities gives plants a deep yellow or orange pigment. A dark green color usually means the plant is loaded with calcium, folate and other important vitamins. So if you want to eat a balanced diet but don't want to spend hours figuring out which foods contain which vitamins and minerals; focus on making every meal you eat as colorful as possible. Try to get all the colors represented.

### 4. Lower Your Fat Intake

Professional groups, such as the American Heart Association, American Diabetes Association, and the United States Department of Agriculture advocate that individuals derive no more than 30% of their calories from fat sources. In addition to diabetes, consuming too much fat, especially saturated fats and cholesterol, will increase the risk of numerous other diseases and disorders such as increased blood cholesterol, heart disease, and various cancers. Diets high in fat will also eventually lead to weight gain and possible obesity.

Clinical studies have demonstrated that a low-fat, plant-based diet will improve insulin resistance, aid in weight loss, and reduce blood sugar, blood pressure, and cholesterol. Diets derived from plants are, by design, very low in saturated fat. This simple diet change could reverse diabetes without portion control or exhausting exercises. **The basic prescription is to simply avoid all animal products (fats and proteins) and eliminate vegetable oils.**

### 5. Don't Overdo Any One Food

No matter how healthy one food might be, you can't eat the same thing forever. Variety is key if you want to make sure you are getting all the nutrition you need from your diet. Plus, certain foods can be unhealthy if you eat too much of it. The goal with any diet is to achieve balance and make sure you get enough of everything you need. Eat only a few select foods and excluding all the others is not the way to go.

### 6.   Do Read the Label

Always, always, always read the label. Better yet, buy food that doesn't need a label because it only has one ingredient: itself. If you're buying tofu, soy milk, or even a bag of mixed greens, read the packaging and make sure it's free of preservatives and other harmful chemicals. Reading the label will not only help you make sure there are no additives, you'll also be able to check for hidden animal products. Some vegetarian products, for example, use dairy or egg in their food. Most of the soy patties you'll find are not vegan friendly. This is yet another reason to avoid processed foods and stick to whole foods that aren't loaded with a million different ingredients. If it's not something you could hypothetically make on your own in the kitchen without calling up a chemistry lab to order some special chemical compounds, you probably shouldn't be eating it anyway.

### 7.   Don't Lose the Balance

Vegans who don't eat fruits and vegetables and stick to vegan-friendly junk food like potato chips and certain candies are widely known as "junk vegans." They become extremely unhealthy because not only are they eating junk food and a lot of fat but they aren't getting a single source of nutrition anywhere in their diet. Don't become a junk vegan.

### 8.   Do Know Your Reasons and Expectations

As with any life decision you make, it's important to know why you are doing it. Do you want to lose weight? Are you concerned about the welfare of animals? Do you want to live a healthier lifestyle? Do you have another reason altogether? You don't have to pick just one reason for doing it. If you have multiple reasons, that's great. It's just important to know them because your personal reasons are what will motivate you and drive you forward. Be specific about your expectations: how much weight do you want to lose or what kind of impact are you hoping to make on the planet? Knowing these things can help you find more ways to achieve your goal. For example, if you are trying to lose weight; combining your vegan diet with a good exercise plan will help you get there even faster. If you are trying to help the environment; setting up a home garden and learning how to grow and make more foods yourself would be the perfect complement to your vegan diet.

### 9. Don't Get Bored

Above all else, do not let yourself get bored with your diet. Constantly try new ingredients, new combinations, and new preparation methods. Sure, you should stick with the ones you really like but always make room for new things and experimentation in your weekly menu. Pick out foods you've never seen before and try a recipe that combines thing you never thought could go together. Even if you don't consider yourself much of a chef, you can still have fun experimenting in the kitchen. Start by finding a lot of different recipes and following them to the letter. After awhile, you'll start to develop a natural sense for what kinds of flavor combinations taste good and what kind of cooking techniques bring out those flavors the best. Let the vegan diet unleash the inner cook in you!

### 10. Do Know When to Cook and When to Go Raw

Within the vegan community, there are some who choose an all raw diet. They do not cook anything. And, while there are certain plants that are better to eat raw; some are actually better for you when cooked. Some trickier ones (like tomatoes) offer different benefits when raw then they do cooked. The reason it's not as easy as going all raw or all cooked is because every vitamin is different. While vitamin C is sensitive to heat and gets destroyed in cooking, A vitamins (including lycopene and beta-carotene) are actually easier for your body to digest after they've been cooked. Here is a quick reference chart you can use for knowing which foods to cook and which to go raw.

It is broken down by nutrient so base your decisions on what the primary vitamin or mineral you are hoping to get from the food is:

| Nutrient | Best Preparation |
|---|---|
| Vitamin A | Cooked |
| Vitamin C | Raw |
| Vitamin D | Go Outside in the Sun! |
| Vitamin E | Cooked |
| Vitamin K | Cooked |
| Vitamin B 6 and B 12 | Cooked |
| Thiamine | Raw or Cooked (below 212° F) |
| Riboflavin | Cooked |
| Niacin | Cooked |
| Biotin | Cooked |
| Pantothenic Acid | Raw |
| Folate | Raw or Low Heat |
| Potassium | Either |
| Chlorine | Either |
| Sodium | Either |
| Calcium | Either |
| Phosphorus | Either |
| Magnesium | Either |
| Zinc | Either |
| Iron | Either |
| Manganese | Either |
| Copper | Either |
| Iodine | Either |
| Selenium | Either |

# 5|
# The 30 Day Vegan Challenge

In this chapter, you'll get all the details you need to take the 30 day vegan challenge and eat a healthy vegan diet with complete nutrition for less than $35 per week. You could cut these costs down even further if you were willing to give up some variety. There are some people who eat vegan diets and only spend $12 per week. They don't sacrifice any nutrition value but they do miss out on variety.

First we will break down the ingredients you'll need to buy. We'll start with your weekly grocery list. This is the main food you'll be eating each week. Many of these items can be found for an even cheaper price if you buy them in bulk so consider bumping this weekly grocery list up to a monthly grocery list to save a few extra bucks.

After the weekly list, you'll get a second list of things that you'll only need to buy once a month (or even less). These are mainly seasonings that you tend to use in very small amounts each day so the large packages last a long time. The final list is a list of supplements. Namely, it lists B12.

Otherwise, the weekly and monthly lists provide you with a full range of nutrients coming from complex carbohydrates that are high in protein and fiber (meaning the meals will keep you feeling full for a long time).

**Weekly Grocery List**

| | |
|---:|---|
| 2 lb brown rice | $1.70 |
| 2 lb black beans | $2.80 |
| 2 lbs lentils | $1.70 |
| 1 lb split peas | $0.65 |
| 1 package pasta noodles | $0.89 |
| 2.5 lbs whole wheat flour | $0.90 |
| 2 packets baking yeast | $0.86 |
| 1 lb carrots | $0.57 |
| 1 ½ lbs onions | $0.70 |
| 10 cloves garlic | $0.30 |
| 1 lb rolled oats | $1.99 |
| 1 bag frozen berries | $1.99 |
| 1 bag frozen spinach | $1.09 |
| 1 bag frozen greens | $1.59 |
| 2 heads broccoli | $1.19 |
| 1 lb apples | $0.76 |
| 1 bunch of bananas | $0.75 |
| 5 lbs potatoes | $3.14 |
| 2 cans tomato paste (6 oz each) | $1.44 |
| 1 jar pasta sauce | $1.99 |
| ½ lb tofu | $1.99 |
| **Total:** | **$29.19** |

**Monthly Grocery List**

| | |
|---:|:---|
| salt* | $0.49 (per pound) |
| pepper* | $3.25 |
| assorted herbs and spices* | ~ $7 |
| coffee (optional)* | $8.98 |
| almond or soy milk (optional) | $1.59 |
| **Total:** | **$12.33** |

This adds about **$3.08** to each week if you calculate the monthly cost. That adjust cost assuming you buy the items with a star (*) next to them only a few times a year (every couple of months or so) which is very likely as you use all of them in limited amounts each day and they come in large packages.

**Supplements**

| | |
|---:|:---|
| B12 Supplement (2,500mcg) | $12.57 |
| **Total:** | **$12.57** |

The supplement looks pricey at first but consider that the B12 will last you about 22 months, making it just $0.14 per week.

Altogether you'll not only have complete nutrition and a good amount of variety, with these items, you can make an enormous variety of foods from fresh baked breads, vegan cookies or pies, vegan pizza, a variety of pasta dishes, chilies, stews, soups, breakfast smoothies, oatmeal with berries, and whatever else you can think up with these ingredients.

All the prices listed here are based on averages. The actual prices of these items in your local grocery stores will, of course, vary. But this should give you a reasonable estimate of what you can expect to spend.

# Additional money saving tips for vegan grocery shopping

- **Always plan ahead**

Plan out every meal you will eat for at least a week in advance. When you do this, you can figure out exactly what you need to buy and how much. This will stop you from letting food go to waste and keep you from making impulse purchases. If it doesn't fit the menu, leave it on the shelf! It's like shopping for clothes: you may have the impulse to get that one pair of shoes but if they don't go with anything in your wardrobe, you know it's a waste of money.

- **Cook ahead**

In addition to planning ahead, you should also cook ahead. You don't always have the time or energy during the week to cook dinner (or even make a quick smoothie for breakfast). But, if you've already got all of your ingredients for the week, you can spend a few hours one day preparing all your meals and then store them in the freezer. Then, during the week, all you'll have to do is pull it out of the freezer, reheat, and enjoy. Complete nutrition and flavor with minimal work! It's like homemade TV dinners except they improve your health instead of destroy it. You can even plan a whole month of meals and then spend one day cooking them and you'll be set for an entire month!

- **Buy frozen instead of fresh**

Fruits and vegetables can get pricey when they are fresh (especially when they are no longer in season). Buy the frozen versions to save money without sacrificing nutrition. Freezing doesn't destroy any nutrition value. Just be careful which ones you reheat (use the chart from chapter 4 to see if it's ok to cook or not). You can also freeze your own fruits and vegetables if you see a great deal on a certain special item. Buy it in bulk and freeze what you won't use that week.

- **Buy seasonal when you buy fresh**

Only buying fresh produce when it's in season will help you save a lot of money. Buying seasonal doesn't mean you have to memorize seasonal harvest times. The seasonal items will usually have the cheapest price per pound. So basically, "buy seasonal" is just another way of saying "buy cheap." Not only will you save money, you'll guarantee variety. Since different produce have different seasons, you're diet will also have a steady rotation so that you don't get sick of eating the same produce all the time.

- **Buy bulk goods when possible**

Another great way to save money is to buy your staple items in bulk. If you know you're going to be eating pounds upon pounds of rice or beans, you might as well opt for the 5 or 10 lbs bag. It'll be a lot cheaper per pound and it will last you a long time. Remember to only buy bulk amounts on food that has a long shelf life. If you can't eat it before it goes bad, there's no reason to buy that much of it.

- **Grow your own food!**

Even if you've got a relatively small plot of soil to grow on (we're talking window planter here), you can still cut costs by planting a few of your favorite, easy to grow veggies. Plant a small herb garden and never buy expensive dried herbs from the store again! Put a tomato plant by your window or plant some carrots in the backyard. There are a lot of great and versatile vegetables that are extremely easy to grow. Having your own garden will save you money, provide you with a regular supply of fresh foods and spices, and give you the perfect hobby to de-stress and relax. Not to mention, gardens look absolutely beautiful and people will admire your green thumb.

You are now fully prepared to begin your 30 day vegan challenge. Start thinking about some recipes that use the ingredients from the list. If you don't consider yourself much of cook, search for some recipes on vegan sites or cookbooks (or ask some of your vegan friends).

You can make slight modifications according to your own tastes and needs but try to remember that you want complex carbs (so no sugar, a lot of starchy foods, and no refined flour) and no oils. Don't go crazy on the healthy fatty foods (avocados, nuts), especially when trying to lose weight. Even if it is healthy fat, there is still such thing as too much of a good thing.

Your most versatile recipe options are to make stews, chilies, or soups. If you have a pressure cooker (or crockpot), experiment with tossing random combinations of veggies, legumes, beans and seasonings to see what you come up with. Learn to make your own bread (that's what the whole wheat flour is on the list for). It is actually really easy. You can make a simple loaf of bread with just flour, yeast, and water. Combine the ingredients, let it rise, toss it in the oven, and you're done.

Not only is homemade bread deceptively easy, it's a thousand times more delicious than any store bought loaf you've ever eaten. It's also a lot healthier as well because there are no unnecessary additives.

The most important thing is to have fun and get creative! So enjoy your new happy, healthy lifestyle and watch the pounds melt away.

# 6|
# Conclusion

At this point, you are hopefully inspired and excited to start on your new journey as a vegan. As you've learned from reading this short book, being vegan can be healthy, exciting, and it can even help you lose tons of weight! By reading through this whole book, you've already taken the first step: getting informed.

Going vegan is more than just a fad diet; it's a whole new way of life that will allow you to get the body you want and to nourish that body fully while living a happier and more stress-free life. You've read through the details of what a vegan diet is; what the many benefits of going vegan are; why the myths you might have heard are wrong; how you can go vegan smartly and healthily; and even gotten a complete plan for taking the 30 day vegan challenge. So what are you waiting for?

Go load up on healthy starches, fruits and veggies and get in the kitchen to start exploring the full potential of your new life as a vegan!

# 7|
# More Groundbreaking Studies

**Don't miss Dr. John McDougalls new FREE Webinars.**

John A. McDougall is an board-certified Internist and best selling author. He claims that degenerative disease can be prevented and treated with a low-fat, whole foods, plant-based diet based on starches (such as potatoes, rice, and corn) which excludes all animal foods and added vegetable oils. His simply practice of using a low-fat, starch-based diet has a broad range of dramatic and lasting health benefits, including dramatic weight loss and reversing serious illnesses, such as heart disease, type-2 diabetes, and arthritis without drugs.

Visit his website at www.drmcdougall.com. Dr. John McDougall also shares how he treats and helps his patients with diet in his free webinars:

# Topic Obesity

## FREE Recorded Webinar:

www.youtube.com/watch?v=OSnHlSv-l1U

*Obesity – Low-Carb Diets Are Dangerous with Dr. McDougall, MD*

More free webinars at: www.drmcdougall.com/webinars

# 8 |

# Bonus-Chapter:
# 7-Day Mealplan Recipes

Eating a whole-foods diet without animal foods and added oils, less salt and sugar, and very few processed foods dramatically improves the health!

The recipes in this book are based on a purely starch-plant based diet (diet based on whole starches, vegetables, and fruits) without added oils. Cheers to you for bidding goodbye to animal products, to processed foods and to oil! Consume only fats that are still in their natural packaging—such as in whole foods.

*The recommended low-fat vegan diet is based on scientific research and recommendations by experts such as Dr. Neal Barnard, T. Collin Campbell, Michael McGregor, and Dr. John McDougall.*

Many times when people make a decision to change their eating habits, the change is short-lived because they get bored or run out of options. This book has been designed to provide you a seven-day meal plan. The recipes within can be mixed and matched to create delicious, healthy, fat-free vegan meals.

The benefits of a vegan, fat-free, plant-based, whole foods diet are vast. Not only will this diet help those who are looking to lose weight, but it is extremely helpful for those suffering from diabetes.

There are recipes for Breakfast, Snacks, Lunch, Dinner and even healthier options for Desserts. **All the recipes are quick and easy.** Even better yet, **each category features two recipes that can be made in fifteen minutes or less or only require five ingredients or less.**

# Monday

## Breakfast: Blueberry Pancakes

**Servings**: 6-8 Pancakes

**Prep Time**: 4 minutes
**Cook Time**: 10 minutes

These pancakes are incredibly easy to make (less than fifteen minutes) and are just as incredibly delicious. You can eat them as-is or add some applesauce as a topping. Whip up a batch for some friends and see if they believe that they are vegan.

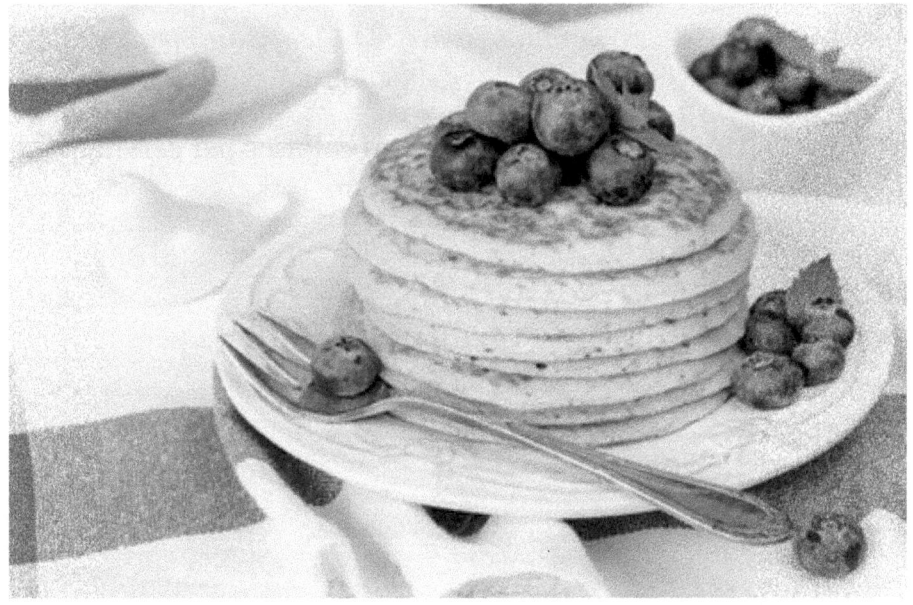

## Ingredients:

- 1 cup whole wheat pastry flower
- 1 tablespoon sugar (you can use your preferred type of

sugar or sweetener)
- 2 tablespoons baking powder
- 1 dash of sea salt
- 1 cup rice milk
- Blueberries to taste

**Instructions:**

1. Set out all your ingredients. Place a pan on the stove over medium heat.
2. Combine all your dry ingredients. Add the rice milk to the mixture and beat until smooth.
3. Spoon the mixture onto the pan. When bubbles begin to appear on the surface, flip the pancake over. Cook until it is brown on both sides.
4. Repeat until all the mixture has been used.

*Tip: These can be made in large batches and frozen. Just pop them in the microwave when you are ready to eat.*

**Nutritional Information:** 400 calories per serving, 65g carbs, 0g fat, 10g protein, 2.4g fiber

# Snack: Vanilla Chia Pudding

**Servings**: 2

**Prep Time**: 5 Minutes
**Cook Time**: 5 Minutes

This recipe will take you a total of ten minutes to prepare ahead of time. Have in your fridge to enjoy a smooth, delicious pudding when a snack attack strikes.

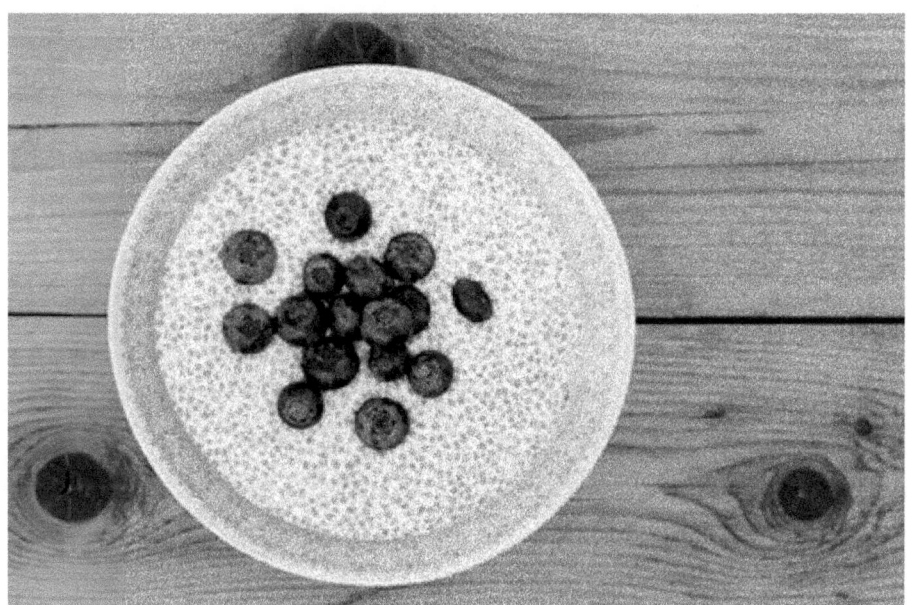

## Ingredients:

- 1 cup Rice Milk
- 4 tablespoons chia seeds
- ½ teaspoon vanilla extract

**Instructions**:

1. Place all of your ingredients into a jar or container that can be shaken.
2. Shake well then place in the refrigerator for at least an hour or overnight.
3. Enjoy.

**Nutritional Information**: 63 calories per serving, 12.6g carbs, 1g fat, 0g protein, 0g fiber

# Lunch: Pesto Pasta

**Servings**: 4

**Prep Time**: 5 Minutes
**Cook Time**: 10 Minutes

I know what you're thinking – *Don't you need oil and cheese for pesto?* The answer is no! Not for this delicious recipe. Enjoy this light and fresh pasta with some vegetables.

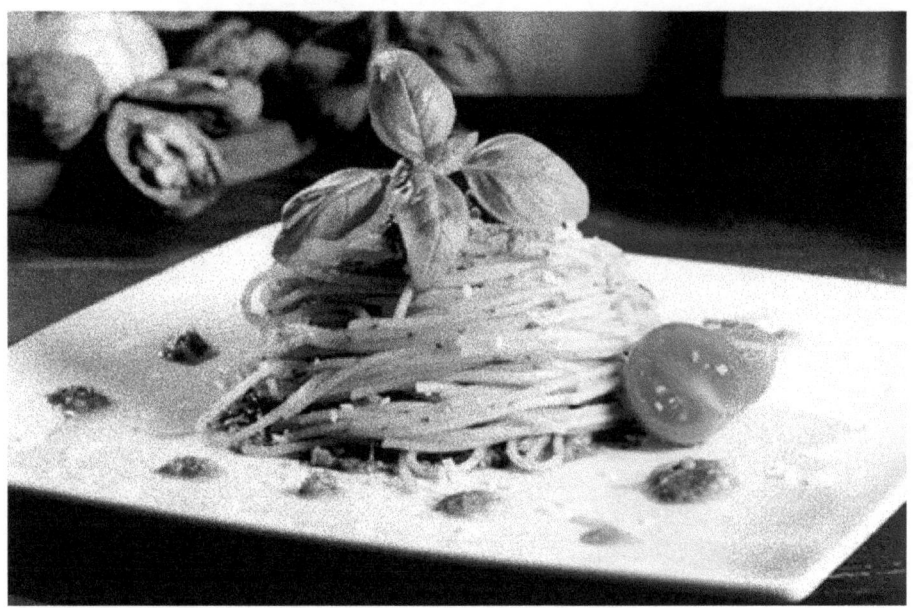

## Ingredients:

- ½ cup water
- ½ cup walnuts
- ½ teaspoon minced fresh garlic (1-2 cloves)
- 1 large bunch fresh basil
- 1 package cooked whole-grain pasta of your choice

**Instructions**:

1. In a food processor, blend all ingredients until smooth. You can use water to thin out as needed.
2. Cook the pasta according to package directions. Once the pasta is cooked, drain.
3. Return the just-cooked pasta to its cooking pot with the heat on medium-low, and add the pesto.
4. Stir until the pasta is completely coated and the pesto is warmed through. Serve while the pesto is still warm.

**Nutritional Information**: 97 calories per serving, 1.7g carbs, 9g fat, 3.8g protein, 1.1g fiber

# Dinner: Black Bean Wrap

**Servings**: 1

**Prep Time**: 5 Minutes
**Cook Time**: 5 Minutes

Let's face it. We don't always want a big elaborate production when it comes to dinner. This wrap will help you serve a dish that is filling and tastes great without all the fuss.

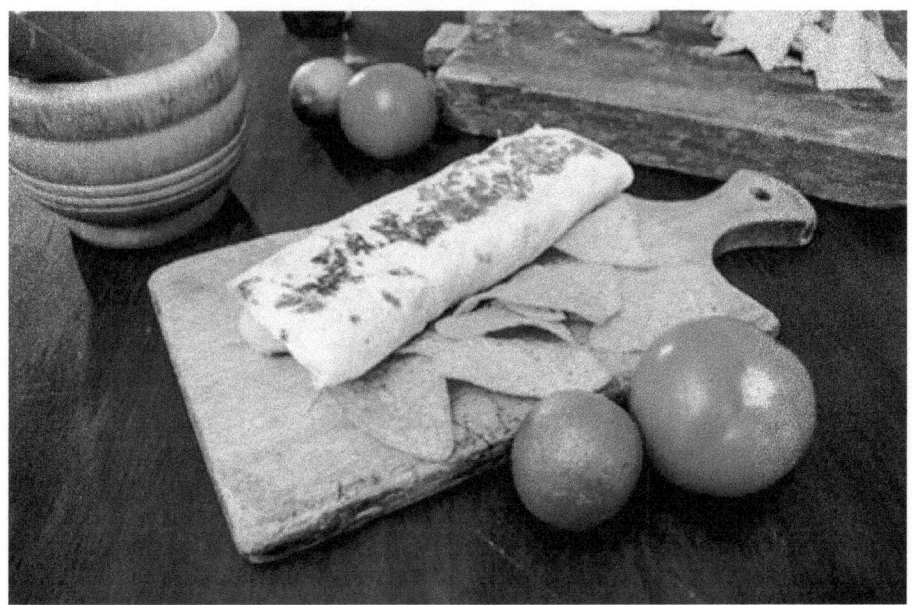

## Ingredients:

- 1 large whole grain tortilla
- ⅓ cup salsa
- ¼ cup black beans
- ¼ cup corn
- ¼ avocado, chopped
- 1 large handful of baby greens
- 2 sprigs of cilantro, chopped

**Instructions:**

1. Warm tortilla using your preferred method.
2. Pour salsa onto the tortilla. It's best to keep to one side in order to make the wrapping part easier.
3. Spread the black beans, corn, and avocado over salsa.
4. Sprinkle the cilantro over the bean mixture and then top with the greens of your choosing.
5. Fold sides of the wrap over the ingredients and then roll from one side to the other. Cut the wrap in half and serve.

**Nutritional Information:** 269 calories per serving, 34.7g carbs, 10g fat, 11g protein, 10g fiber

# Tuesday

## Breakfast: French Toast

**Servings**: 6

**Prep Time**: 5 Minutes
**Cook Time**: 10 Minutes

> Who can resist the aroma of French toast? My recipe will allow you to indulge in this classic breakfast dish and not have all the guilt afterwards or spend all morning making them. Fifteen minutes tops! Oh, and as an added bonus…your kids will be looking for seconds.

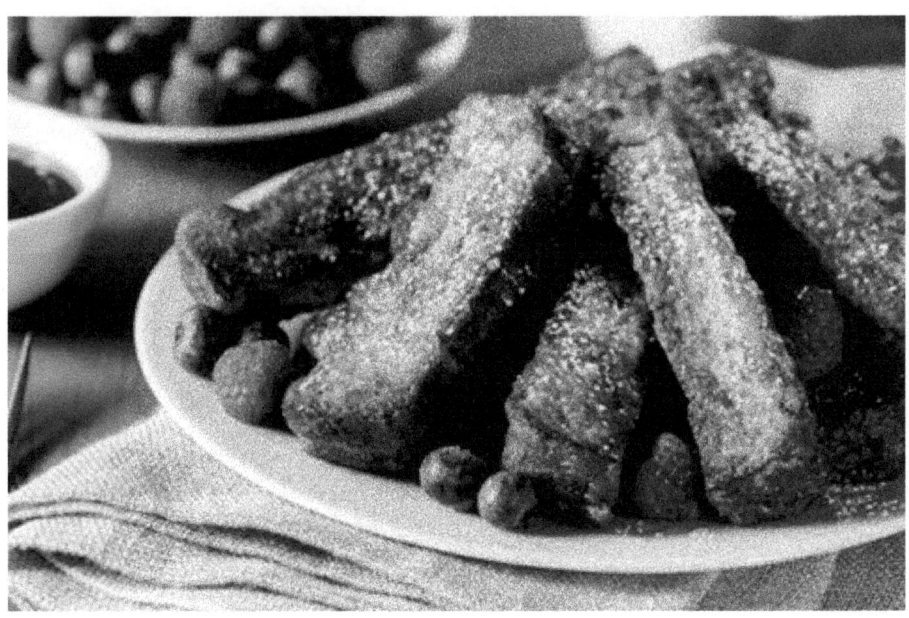

## Ingredients:

- 1 cup original almond smooth milk
- ½ cup orange juice

- 2 tablespoons flour
- 1 tablespoon nutritional yeast
- ½ teaspoon cinnamon
- ¼ teaspoon nutmeg
- 6 slices of whole wheat bread

**Instructions**:

1. Preheat a non-stick skillet over high heat.
2. Add all ingredients to a bowl and mix together.
3. Dip a slice of bread into the mixture and place onto the skillet. Cook for about three minutes on each side.
4. Repeat until you have used all of the mixture and/or bread.
5. Serve and enjoy.

*Tip: If you do not use up all of the mixture, you can store it in the fridge for use at a later time. The mixture will keep for up to five days. Also, if you have extra toasts left over, you can always save them to have later on in the day as a snack. All you have to do is toast them. They are great either plain or with a topping such as bananas or peanut butter.*

**Nutritional Information**: 95 calories per serving, 16.6g carbs, 1.1g fat, 4.8g protein, 2.5g fiber

# Snack: Banana Blueberry Bars

**Servings**: 12 bars

**Prep Time**: 15 Minutes
**Cook Time**: 35 Minutes

These tasty bars make for a wonderful snack. They are full of healthy starches that will provide energy to last you through until your next meal.

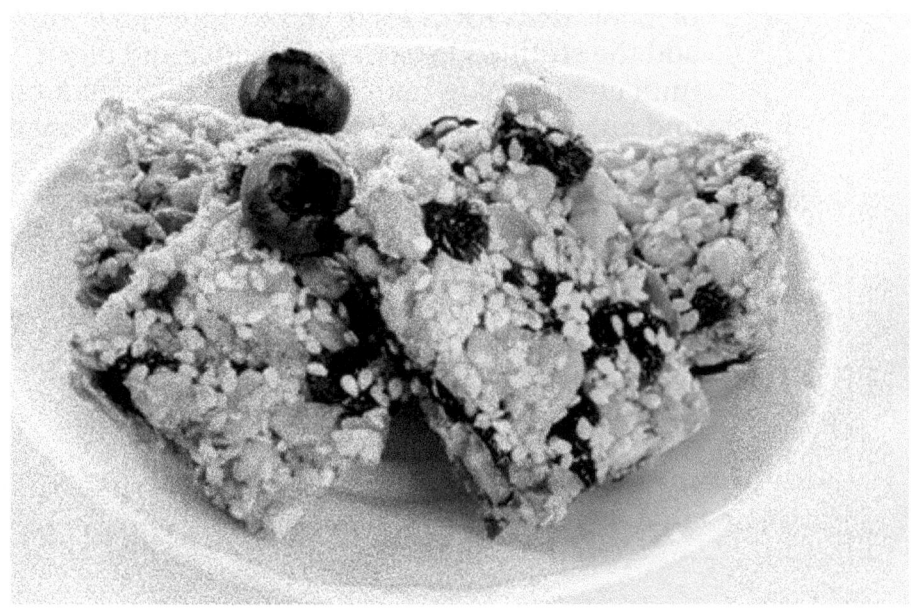

## Ingredients:

- 1 cup dates, pitted and halved
- 1½ cups apple juice
- 1 cup oat flour
- 2 cups rolled oats
- ¾ teaspoon cinnamon
- ¼ teaspoon nutmeg
- 3 bananas
- 1 teaspoon pure vanilla extract

- ½ cup blueberries
- ½ cup walnuts

**Instructions**:

1. Preheat oven to 350°F.
2. Cover a baking pan with parchment paper.
3. Add dates and apple juice into a small bowl and allow the dates to soak for about 10-15 minutes.
4. In a separate bowl, combine flour, oats, cinnamon, and nutmeg. Mix together and set aside.
5. Place the bananas and vanilla extract into a blender. Remove dates from the apple juice and add the strained juice to the blender and blend until creamy. Now add the dates to the blender and pulse a few times until the dates are in small pieces.
6. Pour the banana mixture into bowl with the dry ingredients. Mix all of the ingredients well. Stir in the blueberries and walnuts.
7. Pour the batter into baking pan. Bake at 350°F for 30 minutes. Let cool at room temperature for 5 to 10 minutes before cutting and serving.

**Nutritional Information**: 202 calories per serving, 37.5g carbs, 4g fat, 4.8g protein, 4.7g fiber

# Lunch: Kale, Lemon & Cilantro Sandwich

**Servings**: 2-4

**Prep Time**: 10 Minutes
**Cook Time**: 5 Minutes

This super easy and quick sandwich will have you licking your fingers. Perfect for a quick lunch that will be very filling and satisfying.

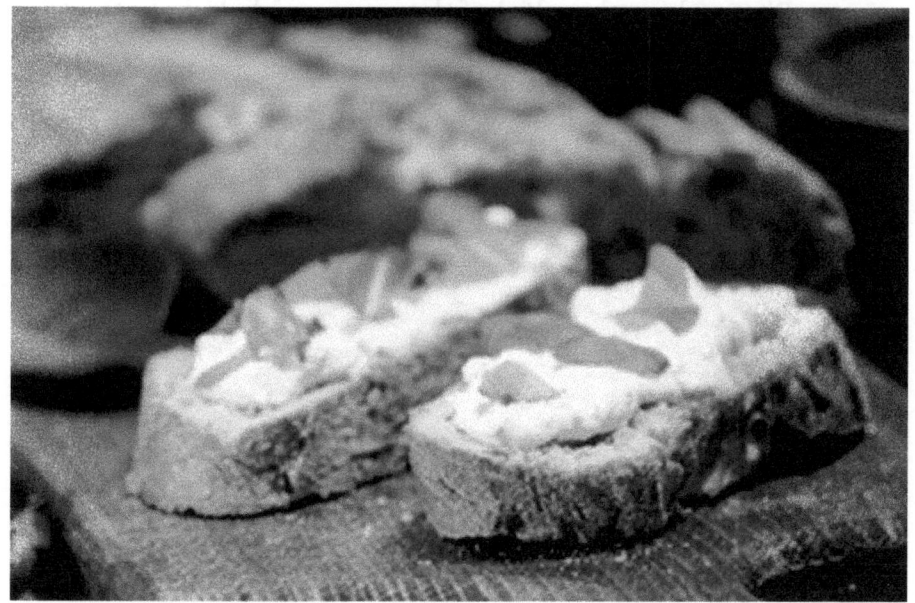

**Ingredients**:

- 1 bunch kale
- 4 slices whole grain bread
- Hummus
- 4 green onions
- ½ bunch cilantro
- 1 lemon sliced thinly into rounds
- Zest of 1 lemon

**Instructions:**

1. Tear kale leaves away from thick stem and chop into bite-size pieces. Place the kale in a pot with about 4 inches of water.
2. Bring to a boil, cover and cook until kale is tender. Check frequently.
3. Spread some hummus onto the bread and then add the green onions, cilantro and lemon rounds on top.
4. Once kale is cooked and drained well, sprinkle with the lemon zest. If you really like lemon, you can squeeze the juice of the remaining lemons on also.
5. Place a large handful of the seasoned kale onto the bread and then top with the other slice.

**Nutritional Information:** 78 calories per serving, 15.3g carbs, 1g fat, 3.8g protein, 2.6g fiber

# Dinner: Quinoa Teriyaki

**Servings**: 4

**Prep Time**: 5 Minutes
**Cook Time**: 10 Minutes

This dish is satisfying and the texture of it is amazing. It's chewy and creamy all in one. It'll be a hit at the dinner table.

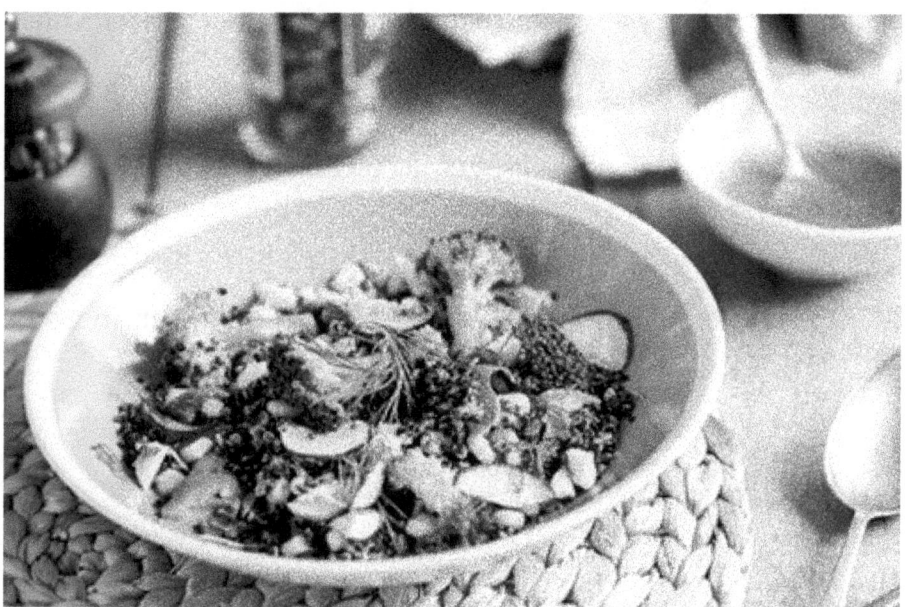

## Ingredients:

- 2 large baked sweet potatoes
- 2 cups cooked quinoa
- ¼ cup water
- 4 cups broccoli florets
- 1 small onion
- 1 avocado
- ½ cup teriyaki sauce

**Instructions**:

1. Add ¼ cup of water to a sauté pan. Add chopped onion, mushrooms and broccoli. Cover and cook on medium high heat for about 10 minutes. Stir occasionally.
2. Warm up the quinoa and sweet potatoes separately in the microwave.
3. When the vegetables are done, add the warmed up quinoa to the sauté pan and stir to mix with vegetables.
4. Serve warmed sweet potatoes into bowls according to servings.
5. Add the quinoa/vegetable mixture right atop of the sweet potatoes and then cover with avocados.
6. Drizzle teriyaki sauce according to taste. Mix lightly and enjoy.

**Nutritional Information**: 486 calories per serving, 72g carbs, 10g fat, 18g protein, 12g fiber

# Wednesday

## Breakfast: Cinnamon Berry Oatmeal

**Servings**: 2

**Prep Time**: 5 Minutes
**Cook Time**: 20 Minutes

There is nothing more comforting than a nice warm bowl of oatmeal in the morning. This oatmeal is especially wonderful because it is naturally sweet and so healthy.

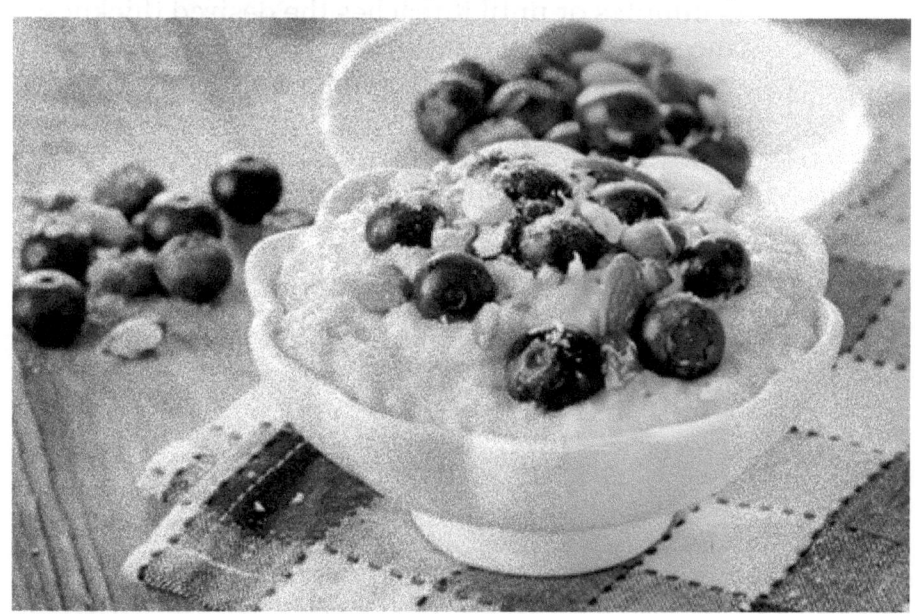

## Ingredients:

- 1 cup water
- 1 teaspoon vanilla extract
- 1/4 teaspoon cinnamon
- 1/2 cup old fashioned rolled oats

- 1/2 cup blueberries (fresh or frozen)
- 2 apples, peeled, cored and diced
- 2 teaspoon chopped walnuts or almonds
- 1 tablespoon ground flax seed

**Instructions**:

1. In a medium saucepan add the water, vanilla and cinnamon and bring to a boil over medium heat.
2. Add the oats and reduce heat to a simmer. Cook for about five minutes.
3. Once the oats have softened, stir in the berries. Continue cooking until all of it is heated through.
4. Remove the saucepan from heat. Cover and let stand 15 minutes or until it reaches the desired thickness. Once the oatmeal has thickened and you are ready to eat, add the apples, nuts and flax.

**Nutritional Information**: 240.7 calories per serving, 40.8g carbs, 6g fat, 17.7g protein, 6.9g fiber

# Snack: Watermelon Salad

**Servings**: 4-6

**Prep Time**: 10 Minutes
**Cook Time**: 0 Minutes

This refreshing, easy to make salad can be either prepared on the spot or ahead of time. It's a great snack to have on hand whenever your sweet tooth strikes.

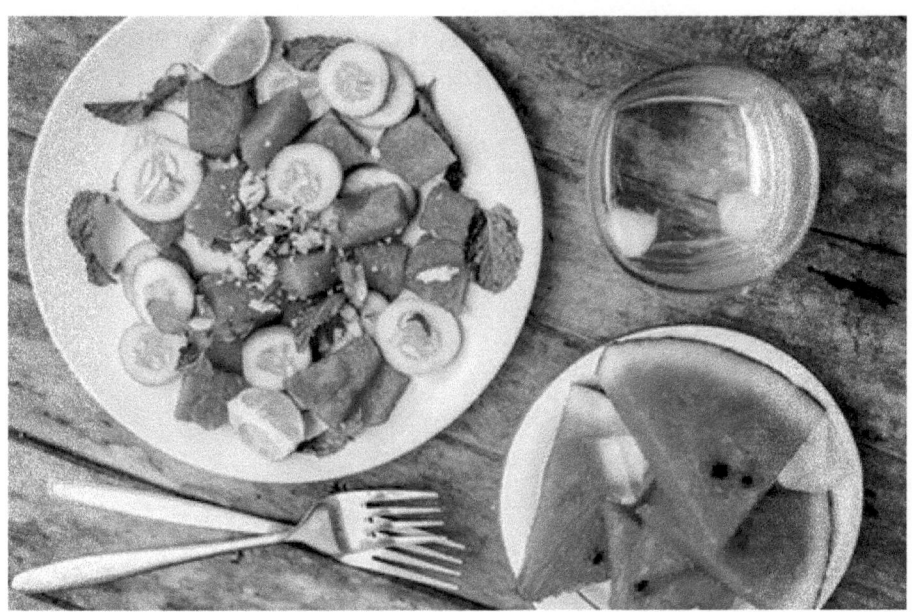

**Ingredients**:

- Half of a Watermelon
- 1 Cucumber
- Chopped mint
- Lime Juice

**Instructions**:

1. Cube and seed the watermelon and cut up the cucumber. The amount of watermelon and cucumber used is entirely up to you.
2. Add fresh mint and lime to taste.

*Tip: If you have too much of this salad left over, do not fret. Throw it into the blender with some ice and turn it into a slushy!*

**Nutritional Information**: 11 calories per serving, 2.6g carbs, 0g fat, 0g protein, 0g fiber

# Lunch: Black Bean Tacos

**Servings**: 8

**Prep Time**: 5 Minutes
**Cook Time**: 10 Minutes

> Who doesn't love a good taco? This recipe will allow you to indulge in some delicious tacos with an amazing cilantro-lime sauce.

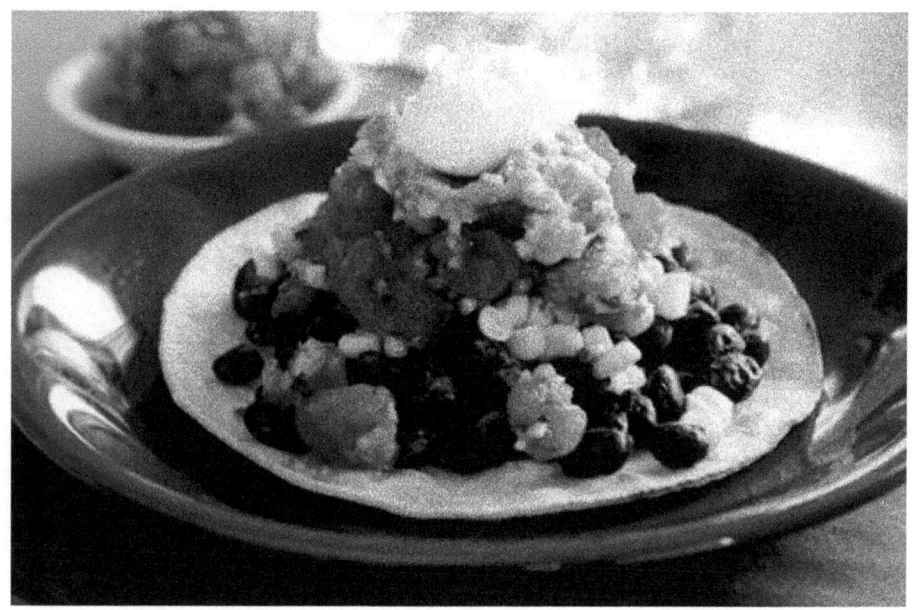

## Ingredients:

- 2 cans of black beans
- 1 cup salsa
- 1 teaspoon cumin
- Corn tortillas
- Toppings of your choice
- ½ avocado
- ¾ cup cilantro (leaves only)
- 1 lime, juiced

- 1 garlic clove
- Pinch of salt

**Instructions**:

1. Begin by preparing the sauce. Add avocado, cilantro, limejuice, garlic and salt to a food processor. Once everything is blended, set aside.
2. Add black beans to a pan over medium heat. Add salsa and cumin. Cook for about five minutes until the beans are heated through.
3. While the beans are heating, warm up your tortillas and prepare your toppings.
4. Assemble your tacos and enjoy!

**Nutritional Information**: 405 calories per serving, 71g carbs, 4g fat, 24g protein, 17.8g fiber

# Dinner: Shepard's Pie

**Servings**: 6

**Prep Time**: 35 Minutes
**Cook Time**: 60 Minutes

This Shepard's pie recipe makes me reminisce of my childhood and when I would sit at the table with my family. Create a new memory for your family or friends with the healthy vegan dish.

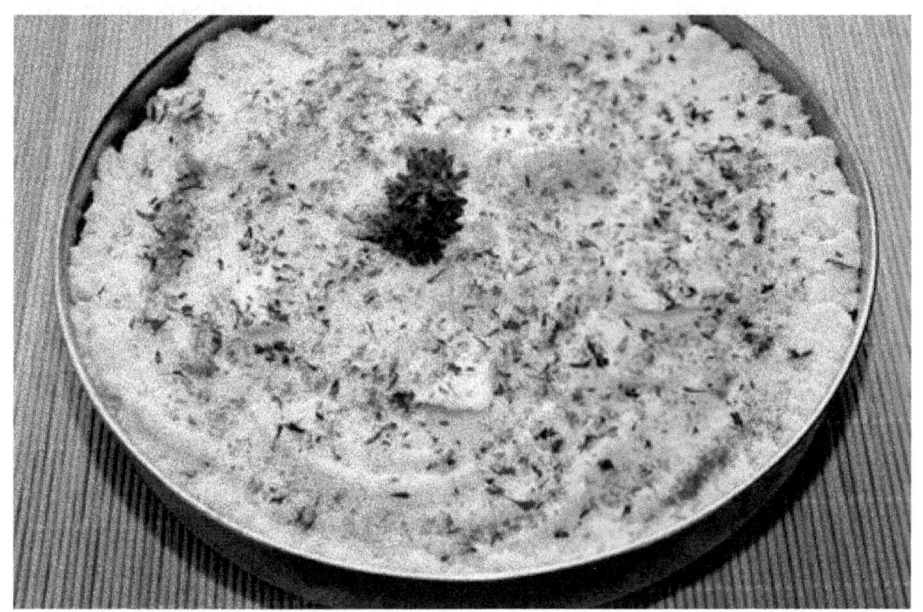

## Ingredients:

- 3 cups veggie broth
- 1 chopped onion
- 1 celery stalk
- 1 green pepper
- ½ teaspoon sage leaves
- 1 tablespoon soy sauce
- 1 carrot

- 1 ½ cups cauliflower florets
- 1 cup cabbage
- 1 cup greens beans
- mix of 2 tablespoons cornstarch & 1/3 cup cold water
- pepper to taste
- 3 cups mashed potatoes

**Instructions**:

1. Preheat oven to 350F.
2. In a large pot, cook ½ cup veggie broth, onion, celery, bell pepper and garlic. Make sure to stir occasionally, for about 4 minutes. Add the sage and soy sauce and stir. Then add the remaining vegetable broth along with the carrots, cauliflower, cabbage and green beans.
3. Bring to a boil and cover, then reduce heat and cook for 20 minutes on low-medium heat.
4. Add the cornstarch mixture and stir until it begins to thicken. Season with pepper to taste.
5. Transfer to a casserole dish and cover vegetable mixture with mashed potatoes. Bake for 30 minutes or until potatoes are slightly browned.

**Nutritional Information**: 127 calories per serving, 25.5g carbs, 1.6g fat, 4g protein, 2g fiber

# Thursday

## Breakfast: Spicy Southern Grits

**Servings**: 2

**Prep Time**: 5 Minutes
**Cook Time**: 15 Minutes

I have to be totally honest and say that the first time I tried grits, many years ago, I hated them. They were bland and the consistency reminded me of what movies depict as "prison food". It wasn't until recently that I tasted this version of grits that I learned what they are really supposed to look and taste like. I guarantee if you've had a not-so-good grit experience in the past, this will totally change your mind.

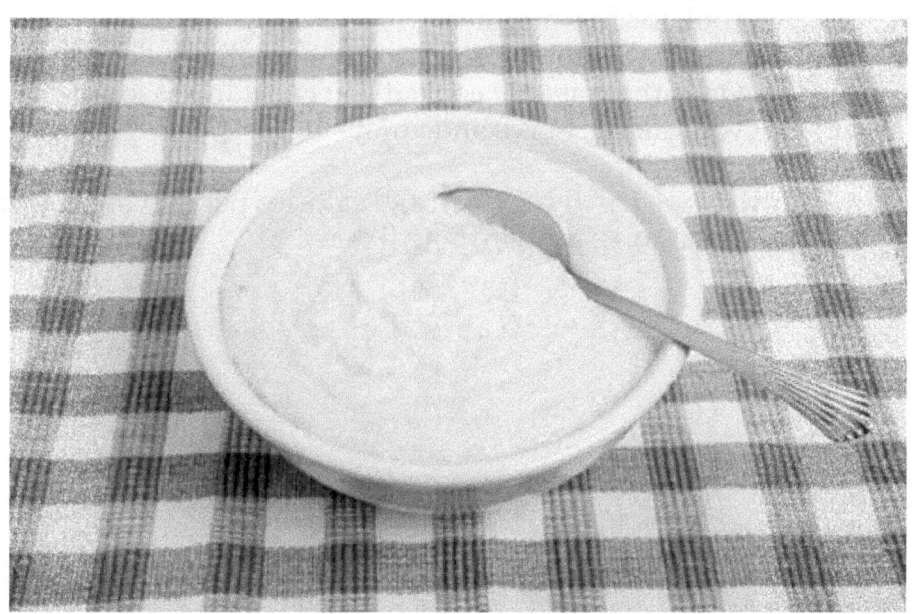

**Ingredients**:

- 1 small yellow onion, diced
- 1 tablespoon garlic, minced
- ¼ cup green chilies, diced
- 1 chipotle pepper, chopped
- 2 cups veggie stock
- ½ cup grits, yellow
- 3 tablespoons nutritional yeast
- ½ lime, juiced

**Instructions**:

1. Sautee the onions, garlic, green chilies and chipotle pepper with 2 tablespoons veggie stock for 5 to 7 minutes.
2. Add the rest of the stock and bring to a boil.
3. Using a whisk, add the grits. Turn the heat to low and cook for five minutes.
4. Stir in the nutritional yeast and the limejuice.
5. Once the grits are cooked you can add seasoning to your liking. Serve and enjoy.

**Nutritional Information**: 137 calories per serving, 24.8g carbs, 3g fat, 9.1g protein, 7.3g fiber

# Snack: Peanut Butter and Jelly Smoothie

**Servings**: 1

**Prep Time**: 5 Minutes
**Cook Time**: 5 Minutes

>This super easy and quick recipe is a great twist on an old favorite. Make this for yourself, for friends or for your whole family.

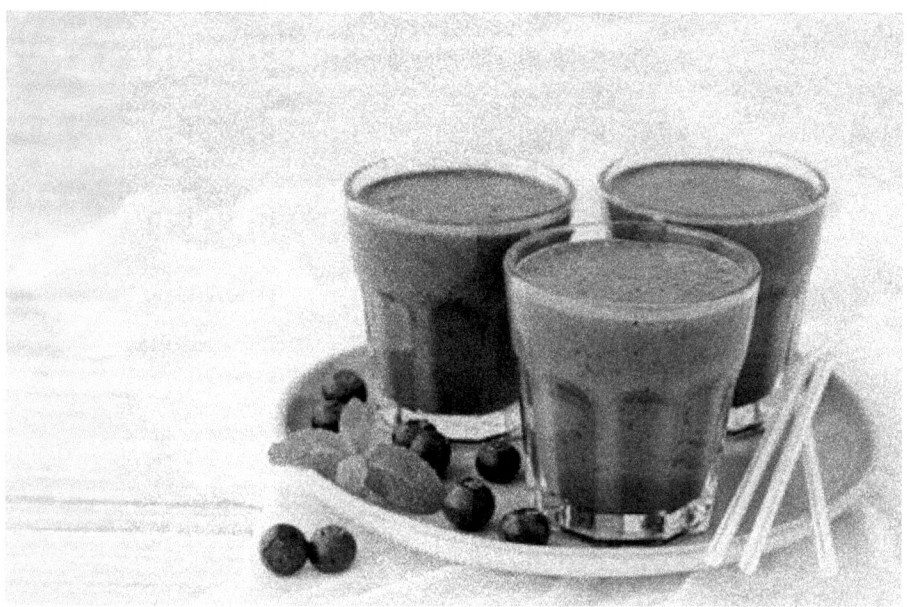

## Ingredients:

- 1 Banana
- 1 cup Raspberries
- 2 Tablespoons Organic Peanut Butter (contains less fat than regular peanut butter)
- 1 ½ cups rice milk of your choosing
- Ice (if using fresh fruits)

**Instructions**:
1. Add all of your ingredients to the blender and blend!
2. Serve and enjoy.

**Nutritional Information**: 349 calories per serving, 78.9g carbs, 4.2g fat, 3.4g protein, 11g fiber

# Lunch: Black Beans and Rice

**Servings**: 5

**Prep Time**: 15 Minutes
**Cook Time**: 10 Minutes

This dish is as basic as they come, but the flavor will tell a whole different story. Prepare this for your family or impress some friends.

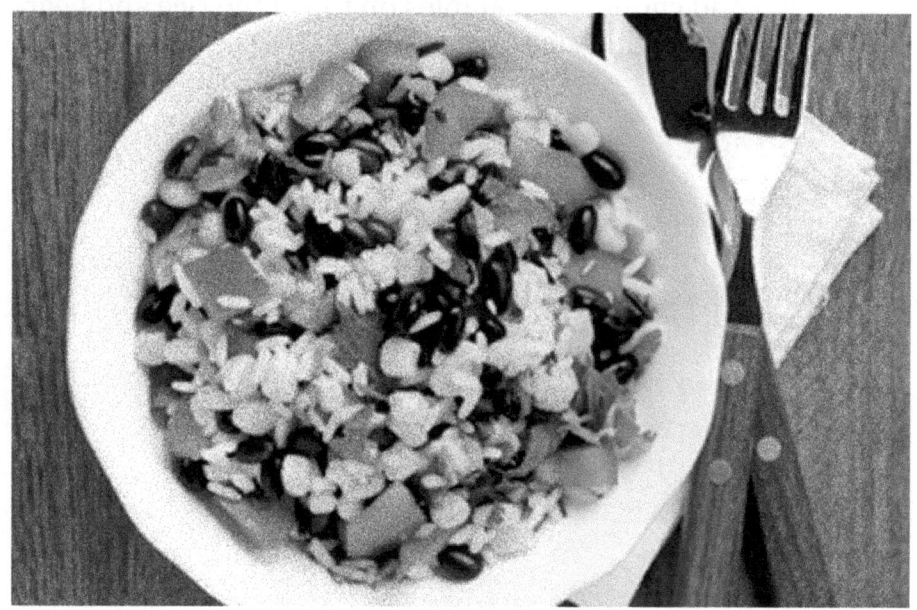

**Ingredients**:

- 2 cans of black beans
- 1 cup veggie stock
- 1 tablespoon Liquid Aminos
- 1 teaspoon red chili powder
- 2 chopped tomatoes
- 3 chopped green onions
- 1 cup corn
- 2 chopped and seeded green peppers

- 1 bunch cilantro leaves
- 1 avocado
- 3 cups cooked rice
- Salsa to taste

**Instructions**:

1. Heat the beans with about 2 cups of water, the liquid aminos and chili powder.
2. Serve the rice onto plates. Ladle the beans over the rice according to taste.
3. Add chopped vegetables on top of the rice and beans.
4. Cover with salsa to taste.

*Tip: You can use pinto or kidney beans in place of black beans.*

**Nutritional Information**: 703 calories per serving, 119g carbs, 10g fat, 39g protein, 30.3g fiber

# Dinner: Vegetable Pasta

**Servings**: 4-6

**Prep Time**: 15 Minutes
**Cook Time**: 15 Minutes

This one-pot pasta recipe will be the recipe that will keep on giving. Why? Substitute different vegetables and pasta sauce every time you make it and will be like a whole new dish each time.

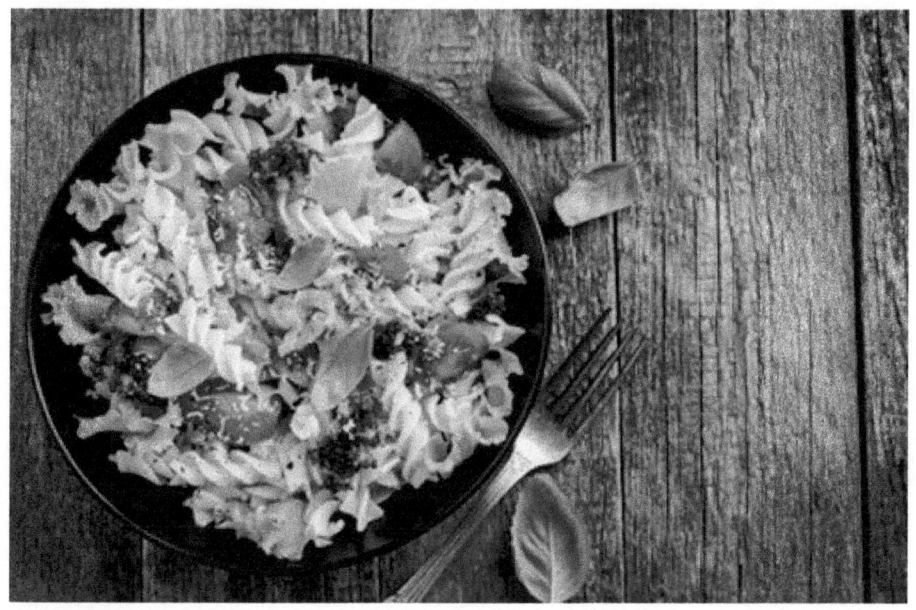

## Ingredients:

- 1 lb. pasta (preferably wholegrain)
- 2 cups broccoli florets
- bunch of spinach
- cherry tomatoes
- 1 jar of your favorite pasta sauce

**Instructions**:
1. Cook pasta in a large pot according to package directions.
2. In a separate pot, cook vegetables according to preferred softness.
3. Drain the pasta and vegetables then add everything into one pot and mix with pasta sauce.

**Nutritional Information**: 245 calories per serving, 46.2g carbs, 2g fat, 11g protein, 2g fiber

# Friday

## Breakfast: Blueberry Muffins

**Servings**: 1 dozen

**Prep Time**: 30 Minutes
**Cook Time**: 30 Minutes

Let's face it. We don't always have the time or desire to sit down and eat breakfast, even if it is the most important meal of the day. Cook up a batch of these muffins ahead of time and have a delicious, quick option you can have on those on-the-go days.

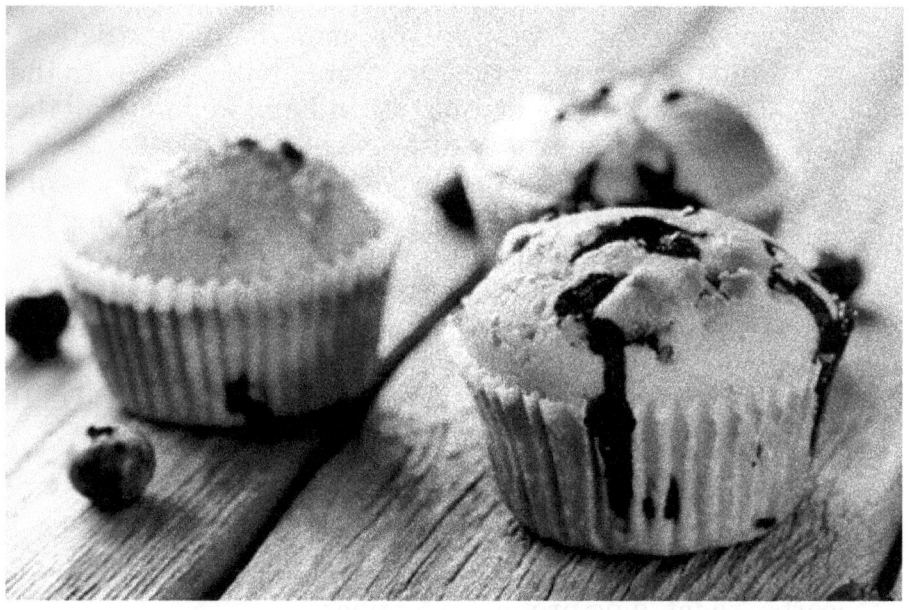

### Ingredients:

- 12 dates, pitted and chopped
- 1 cup almond milk

- 1½ cups old-fashioned rolled oats
- ¾ cup dry millet
- 2 teaspoons baking powder
- ½ teaspoon ground cardamom
- ½ cup applesauce
- 1 teaspoon lemon zest, packed
- 1 cup blueberries

**Instructions:**

1. Preheat your oven to 350. Mix the chopped dates and the almond milk in a small bowl and set aside for about 15 to 20 minutes so that the dates can soften.
2. Using your blender, grind the oats and millet into a flour consistency. Mix the flour, baking powder and cardamom in a separate bowl and stir all the ingredients together.
3. Pour the dates and almond milk mixture into the blender and blend until it is smooth. Add the date mixture to the bowl of dry ingredients along with the applesauce and lemon zest, and mix well until all the dry ingredients have disappeared.
4. Gently fold in the blueberries. Once everything is mixed together, spoon the batter into muffin pan, filling each muffin cup about halfway full.
5. Bake the muffins for 25 to 30 minutes. You will know the muffins are ready when the tops begin to brown and cracks show up on the muffin top. You could also use the "toothpick test" to see if they are ready. Let the muffins cool for at least 15-20 minutes before removing.

**Nutritional Information:** 129 calories per serving, 19.8g carbs, 5g fat, 2.2g protein, 2.6g fiber

# Snack: Apple Cookies (A healthier cookie option)

**Servings**: 2

**Prep Time**: 5 Minutes
**Cook Time**: 0 Minutes

Next time that you are craving a snack, make this easy and delicious recipe. Once again, this one is great for the kids, and they won't even realize they are eating a healthier option.

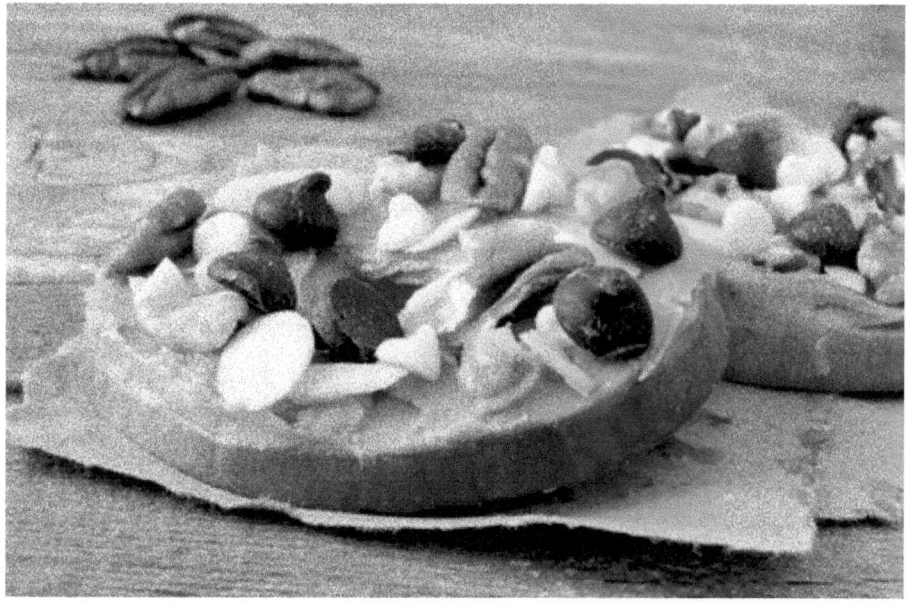

## Ingredients:

- 1 apple, sliced and cored
- 2 tablespoons organic peanut butter
- Mini dairy-free chocolate chips

**Instructions**:

>Spread peanut butter on top of the apple slices. Next sprinkle each slice with chocolate chips. Serve and enjoy!

*Tip: You can substitute the chocolate chips with shredded coconut, raisins, almonds or any other of your favorite toppings.*

**Nutritional Information**: 47 calories per serving, 12.6g carbs, 0.2g fat, 0.2g protein, 2.2g fiber

# Lunch: Mac n' Cheese

**Servings**: 6

**Prep Time**: 20 Minutes
**Cook Time**: 20 Minutes

Nothing says all-American like a nice warm bowl of Mac n' Cheese. Well, now even us Vegans can enjoy this all-time favorite.

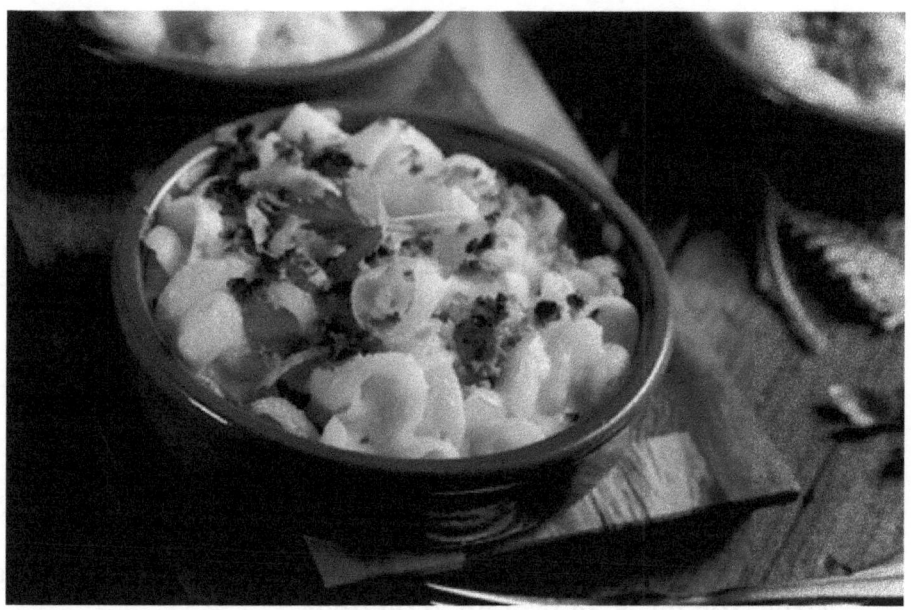

**Ingredients**:

- 1½ cups raw cashews
- 3 tablespoons lemon juice
- ¾ cup water
- 1½ teaspoon sea salt
- ¼ cup nutritional yeast
- ½ teaspoon chili powder
- ½ clove garlic
- pinch of turmeric

- pinch of cayenne pepper
- ½ teaspoon Dijon mustard
- 8 oz. of elbow or shell pasta of choice

**Instructions**:

1. Preheat the oven to 350F. Start boiling some water to prepare your pasta. Cook according to package directions.
2. Add the cashews into a blender and blend until they are finely ground. Once the cashews have been processed and are the correct consistency, add the rest of the ingredients and blend until you have a thick smooth consistency.
3. By this point, your pasta should be ready or very close to it. Once it is cooked to your liking, drain and rinse it. Once drained, return it to the pot. Now add the "cheese sauce" and mix well with the pasta. Let it sit on low heat for a couple of minutes to heat the sauce through.
4. Serve while hot and enjoy!

*Tip: You can also add veggies to this dish. Some delish sautéed broccoli would make this dish even more amazing.*

**Nutritional Information**: 224 calories per serving, 14.7g carbs, 10g fat, 8.4g protein, 2.9g fiber

# Dinner: Chickpea Chili

**Servings**: 6

**Prep Time**: 35 Minutes
**Cook Time**: 45 Minutes

This chili is a great comfort dish everyone will love. It will be worth the wait, guaranteed.

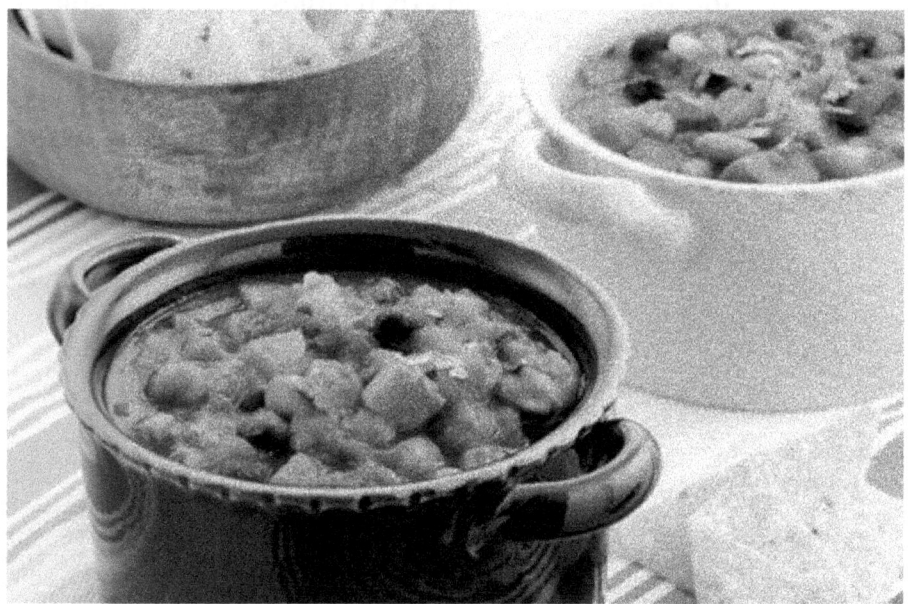

## Ingredients:

- 1 diced onion
- 2 garlic cloves, minced
- 1 diced jalapeño
- 2 cans chickpeas
- 1 can of creamy white bean of choice
- 1 can diced green chiles (=chilies)
- 1½ teaspoon cumin
- 1 teaspoon dried thyme
- ¼ teaspoon pepper

- 1 teaspoon oregano
- 1 teaspoon smoked paprika
- 1 teaspoon chili powder
- 3 cups vegetable stock
- 1 cup corn

**Instructions**:

1. In a pot sauté the onion, garlic and jalapeño over medium heat for 5 minutes.
2. Add the beans, diced green chiles and all the spices. Mix everything well. Stir in the broth and simmer for 20-30 minutes.
3. Add the corn and let simmer for about 2-3 minutes longer.
4. Serve hot with your favorite toppings.

**Nutritional Information**: 35 calories per serving, 8g carbs, 0.5g fat, 1.2g protein, 1.5g fiber

# Saturday

## Breakfast: Breakfast Cookies

**Servings**: 12

**Prep Time**: 10 Minutes
**Cook Time**: 25 Minutes

So, you've been working hard all week to eat healthy. You deserve a treat, don't you? These breakfast cookies are exactly what you need. They are full of good stuff, so there will be no room for guilt after eating these.

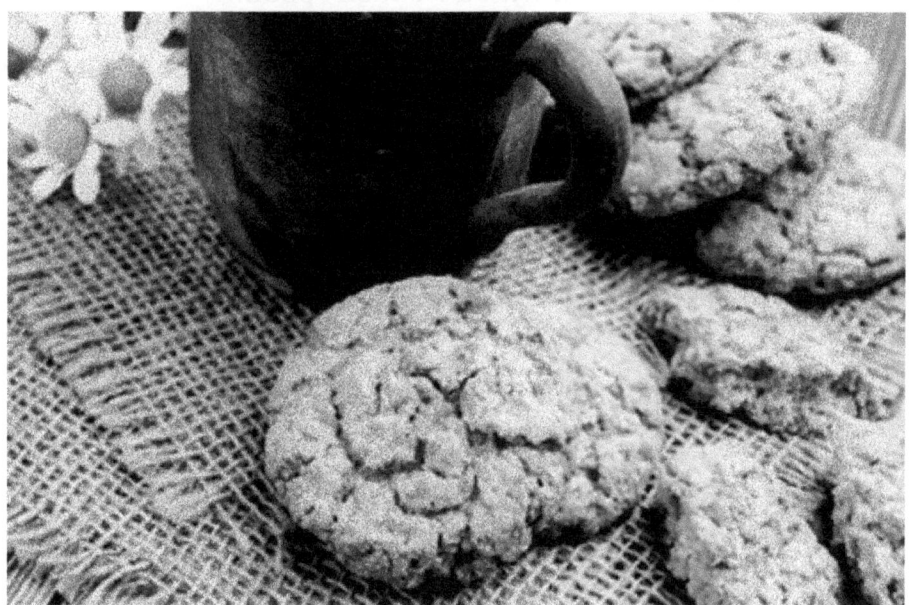

**Ingredients**:

- ¼ cup unsweetened applesauce
- 2 tablespoons chia seeds
- ½ cup date paste
- 1 teaspoon vanilla extract
- 2 ripe bananas, mashed

- 2 tablespoons fine chopped walnuts
- 1 cup rolled oats
- ½ cup unbleached flour
- ½ teaspoon baking soda

**Instructions**:

1. Preheat oven to 350 degrees.
2. Combine the applesauce, chia seeds, date paste and vanilla and bananas into a bowl and mix until smooth. Set the bowl aside so that the chia seeds can start to gel.
3. In a separate bowl, combine the walnuts and the dry ingredients. Combine the wet ingredients into this mix. Mix well with a wooden spoon.
4. Scoop the cookies onto the baking sheet. With a spatula or a knife, flatten the cookies to your desired thickness. Thicker cookies will be chewier.
5. Place in oven and bake for 23-25 minutes. Once they are ready, remove and let cool before serving.

***Tip**: These can be stored in an airtight container or Ziploc and frozen.*

**Nutritional Information**: 92 calories per serving, 18.7g carbs, 1g fat, 2.1g protein, 1.7g fiber

# Snack: Strawberry Banana Popsicles

**Servings**: 6

**Prep Time**: 10 Minutes

Yummy, clean-eating popsicles made with only 3 ingredients? Where can I sign up? Trust me, you will have a hard time eating just one!

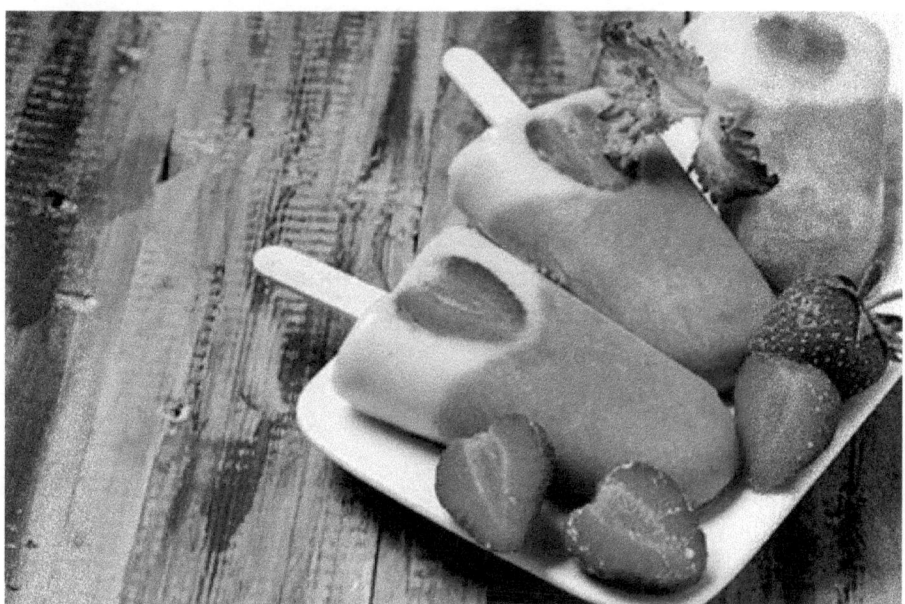

## Ingredients:

- 1 large ripe banana
- 12 large strawberries, sliced in half
- ½ cup fruit juice of your choice

*Note: You will need a popsicle mold and popsicle sticks for this recipe.*

**Instructions**:

1. Add all of the ingredients into a blender and blend on high speed until smooth.
2. Pour the mixture into a popsicle mold. Add your popsicle sticks. (If your mold does not have slots for these you will have to freeze mixture for a couple of hours then insert the sticks and continue freezing.)
3. Let popsicles freeze overnight. Once you are ready to serve you can run the molds under warm water help remove the popsicles. Enjoy!

*Tip: Taste your mixture before freezing so that you can adjust the flavor if necessary.*

**Nutritional Information**: 32 calories per serving, 7.9g carbs, 0.2g fat, 0.5g protein, 1.3g fiber

# Lunch: Black Bean Veggie Burger

**Servings**: 6

**Prep Time**: 15 Minutes
**Cook Time**: 35 Minutes

I'm sure you would agree that no collection of vegan recipes would be complete without a vegan burger recipe. Well, here we are giving you a great burger you can cook up in no time.

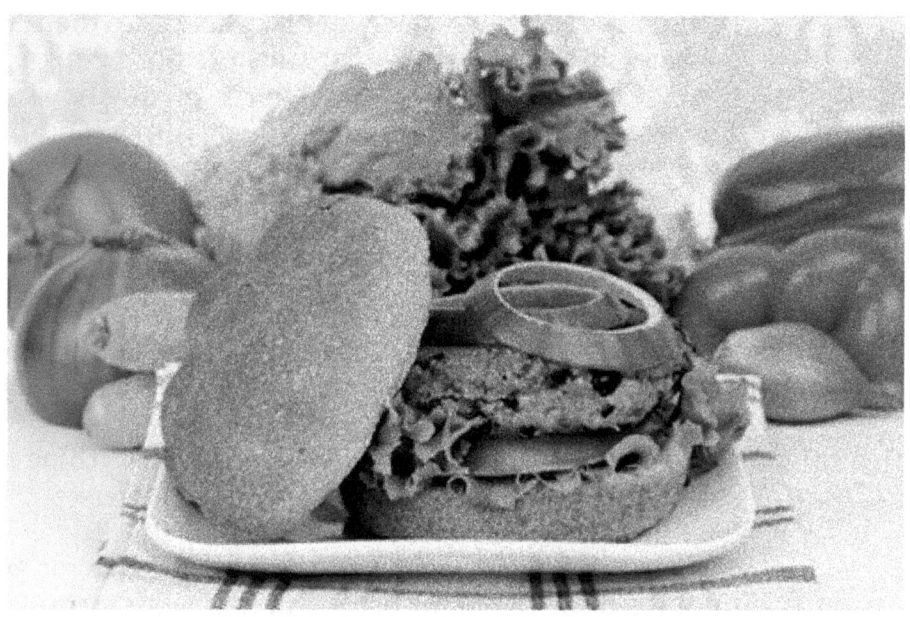

## Ingredients:

- 1 red bell pepper
- 5 small red potatoes
- 2 cans black beans, drained and rinsed
- ¾ cup smooth salsa
- 2 teaspoons chili powder
- 1 teaspoon ground cumin
- ¼ cup medium grind coarse cornmeal

**Instructions**:
1. Preheat oven to 400 degrees.
2. Chop your bell pepper. Make sure to cut it into small pieces so that it will mix easily with the burger batter. Place them onto a sheet pan lined with parchment paper and roast in the oven for about 10 minutes.
3. Peel the potatoes and wrap them in plastic. Cook them in the microwave until they are tender. Alternately, you could roast them, but do NOT boil as boiling will make the burgers mushy. Mash the cooked potatoes and measure out 1 tightly packed cup. Set this aside.
4. Drain and rinse your black beans. Make sure there is no excess water on the beans. Measure out 1 cup of the black beans and place into a large mixing bowl. The rest of the beans should be placed into a food processor. Add the potatoes to the processor as well. Pulse until you have a sticky, thick mashed paste. It should only take a few pulses.
5. Add this mixture to the bowl of extra beans.
6. In a separate small bowl, combine the salsa, chili powder, and cumin and mix well. Pour the salsa mixture over the bowl of beans and potatoes and add the cooked bell pepper.
7. Mix all of the ingredients together until everything is combined well and you have a thick, sticky paste.
8. Lastly, mix the cornmeal into the batter until combined well. Place the batter into the fridge for 30 minutes prior to baking. This will help with forming the patties later on.
9. After chilling, form 6 patties and place them on a sheet pan lined with parchment paper.
10. Bake at 375 degrees for 25 minutes. Remove the pan and using a thin metal spatula carefully flip them. After you have flipped all 6 patties, cook for additional 10 minutes.
11. Remove the patties from the oven and let cool while you prepare your patties and the toppings you will use.

**Nutritional Information:** 616 calories per serving, 117.6g carbs, 2.7g fat, 34g protein, 25.6g fiber

# Dinner: Lasagna Rolls

**Servings**: 5

**Prep Time**: 10 Minutes
**Cook Time**: 25 Minutes

Lasagna is one of my favorite dinner dishes. It's great for dinner parties or for a few guests. Cook up a batch and serve this at your next get-together or for a simple family meal.

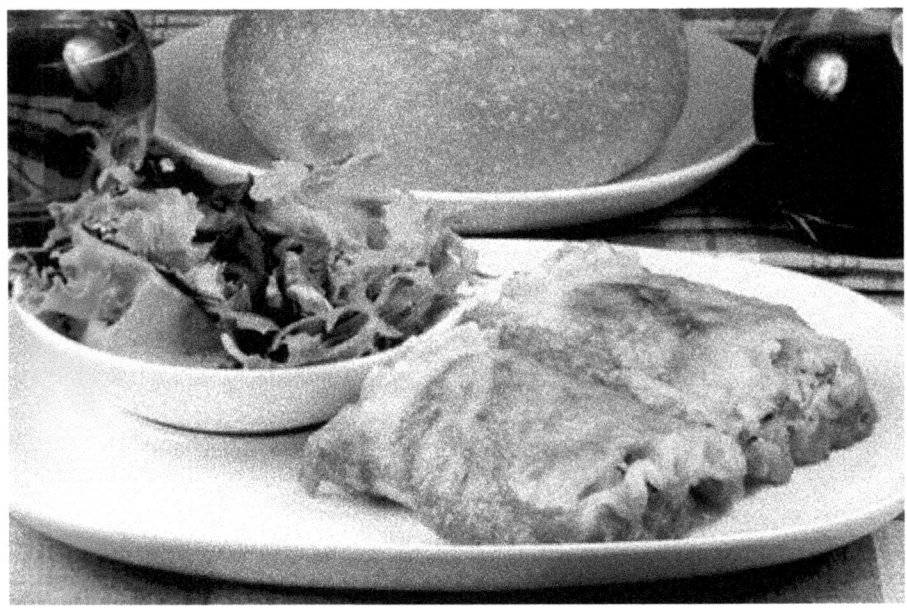

## Ingredients:

- lasagna noodles
- 2 ripe avocados
- 2 tablespoons vegan Parmesan
- ¼ teaspoon garlic powder
- 2 teaspoon basil
- 1/3 cup chopped baby spinach leaves
- 1 tablespoon parsley
- 6 grape tomatoes

- pepper to taste
- ½ cup sauce

**Instructions**:

1. Preheat oven to 350F.
2. Cook about 5 lasagna noodles according to package directions.
3. Combine to avocado, Parmesan, garlic powder, basil, spinach, parsley, tomatoes and pepper. Mix all these ingredients until they are well combined.
4. In a baking dish, cover the bottom with marinara sauce.
5. Take one lasagna noodle and place it on a clean flat surface. Spread some of the mixture across the entire length of the noodle. Roll up the noodle and place upright into the baking dish. Repeat this for all the noodles.
6. Cover the dish with aluminum foil and bake for 20 minutes.

**Nutritional Information**: 281 calories per serving, 23g carbs, 17g fat, 5g protein, 9g fiber

# Sunday

## Breakfast: Breakfast Tortillas

**Servings**: 6-8

**Prep Time**: 10 Minutes
**Cook Time**: 10 Minutes

Here's a little fancier dish that you can serve occasionally at home, or make for guests. It is very filling and something different to change things up a bit.

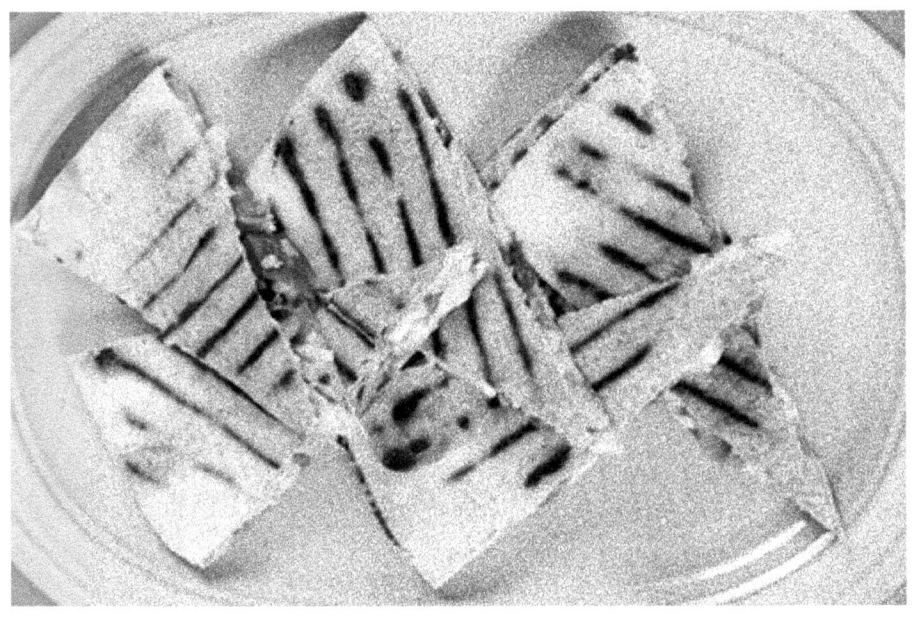

### Ingredients:

- 2 cups packed spinach
- 2 cups cooked brown rice
- 1 cup frozen corn kernels
- ½ cup salsa

- 6 to 8 whole wheat or corn tortillas

**Instructions**:

1. Place the spinach in a saucepan. Make sure that the leaves are wet. Cook for about two minutes, or until it is just wilted. Remove from the saucepan and drain well.
2. Place the brown rice, corn, and salsa in the saucepan. Cook until heated through and then stir in the spinach.
3. Once everything is cooked spoon some of the mixture onto each tortilla and roll.

**Nutritional Information**: 234 calories per serving, 49.5g carbs, 2g fat, 5.6g protein, 3.7g fiber

# Snack: Baked Sweet Potato Chips

**Servings**: 1-2

**Prep Time**: 15 Minutes
**Cook Time**: 12 Minutes

The perfect snack! These oil-free and easy to prepare chips will be just what you need to satisfy your craving for salty and crunchy.

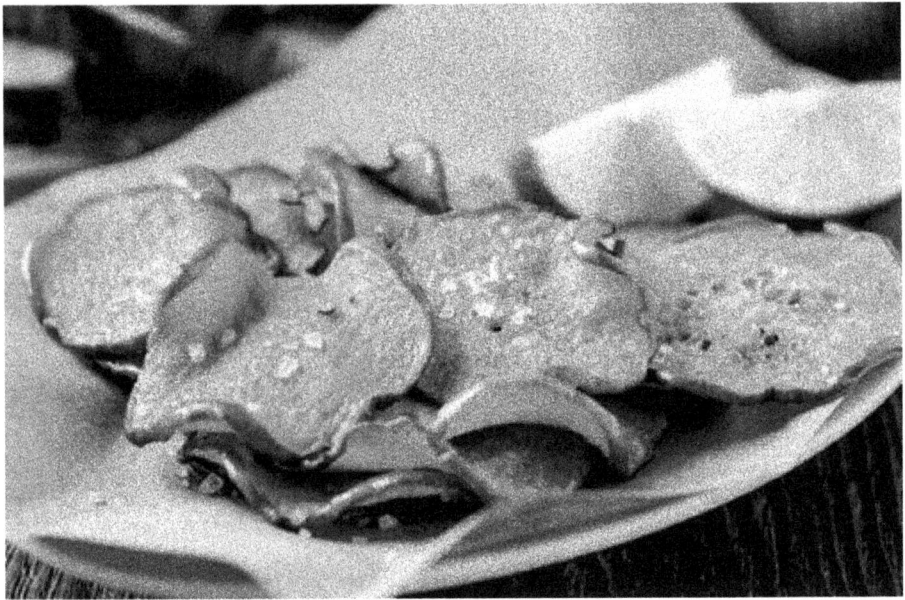

### Ingredients:

- Large sweet potato
- Fine sea salt, to taste
- Seasonings of choice

### Instructions:

1. Preheat oven to 400F.

2. Slice the potato into really thin slices, with or without the skin. (The use of a mandolin will be your best option, but it is not the only option.)
3. Prepare a baking sheet lined with parchment paper and arrange the slices in a single layer.
4. Sprinkle with sea salt and any other seasoning you have chosen.
5. Bake in the oven for 10 minutes. Flip each slice and continue to bake for another 2-3 minutes. Make sure to keep an eye on them because they will burn easily.

**Nutritional Information**: 163 calories per serving, 37.3g carbs, 0.3g fat, 3.6g protein, 6g fiber

# Lunch: Tomato Soup

**Servings**: varies depending on use

**Prep Time**: 20 Minutes
**Cook Time**: 20 Minutes

To round up our delicious lunch section, we are offering you a wonderful and easy-to-prepare soup. This soup is great year round.

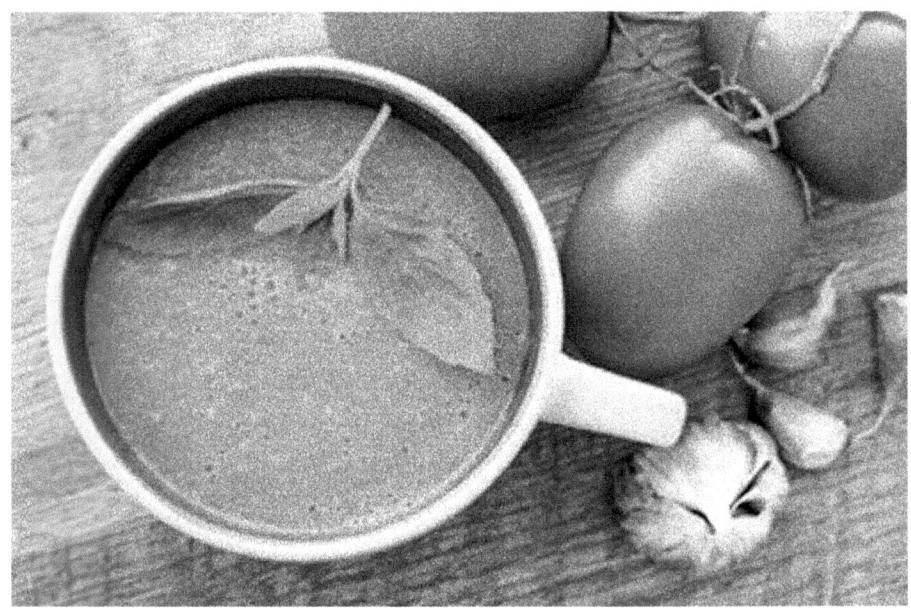

### Ingredients:

- 1 onion, diced
- 2 garlic cloves, minced
- 2 tablespoons water
- 4 lbs. ripe tomatoes
- 1 cup vegetable broth
- Cilantro for garnish

**Instructions:**

1. Prepare a large pot with water and add the diced onion and minced garlic. Cook until they are soft, adding water as necessary.
2. Add the tomatoes (which should be peeled, seeded, and chopped) and broth to the pot. Bring to a boil then reduce heat and simmer for about 15 minutes.
3. Once this is cooked, add to a blender and puree.
4. Serve the soup and garnish with some cilantro or other herb of your choosing.

**Nutritional Information:** 139 calories per serving, 27.9g carbs, 1.7g fat, 7.5g protein, 8.1g fiber

# Dinner: Tortilla Casserole

**Servings**: 6

**Prep Time**: 15 Minutes
**Cook Time**: 15 Minutes

This casserole is a one-dish wonder. You can have dinner ready on the table in 30 minutes! Great for those long days.

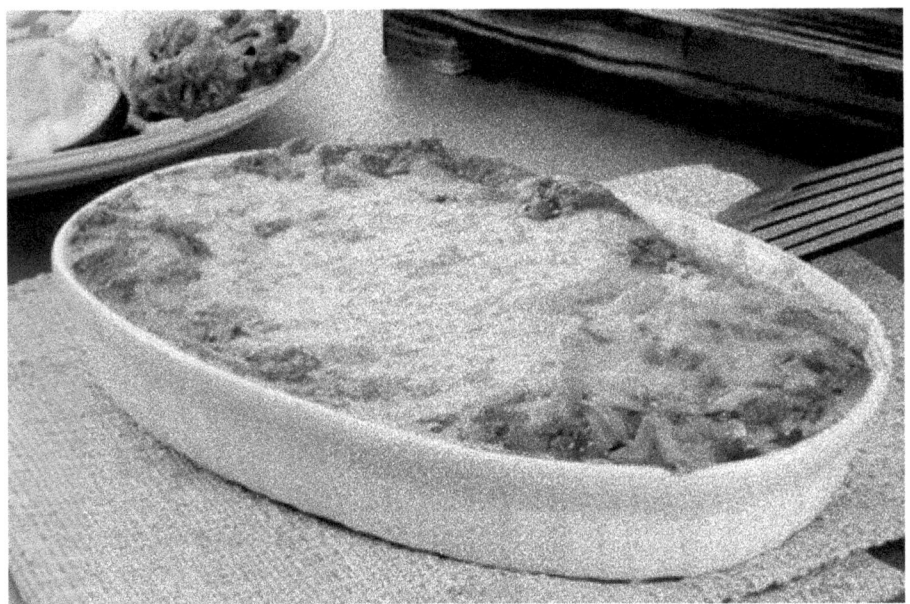

**Ingredients**:

- 1 can black beans, drained and rinsed
- 1 can diced tomatoes
- 1 can chopped mild green chilies
- 2 cups corn kernels
- 1 bunch scallions, chopped
- 1 teaspoon chili powder
- 1 teaspoon ground cumin
- ½ teaspoon dried oregano
- 12 corn tortillas

- 2 cups vegan cheese
- Salsa

**Instructions**:

1. Preheat oven to 400° F.
2. Combine beans, tomatoes, chilies, corn, scallions, chili powder, cumin, and oregano in a bowl.
3. Line the bottom of a casserole dish with 6 tortillas, allowing them to overlap in the middle. Scoop on half of the bean mixture and sprinkle on half of the cheese. Add another layer of tortillas as you did before and add the rest of the bean mixture and the rest of the cheese.
4. Bake in the oven for 12-15 minutes.
5. Cut into squares and serve with your favorite salsa.

**Nutritional Information**: 396 calories per serving, 77g carbs, 2.9g fat, 19g protein, 15.6g fiber

# Dessert – Healthier Options

## Peach Cobbler

**Servings**: 1

**Prep Time**: 5 Minutes
**Cook Time**: 2 Minutes

This peach cobbler is so easy it will take you all of seven minutes to make. Break this out after a great dinner and everyone will think you slaved all day making this treat.

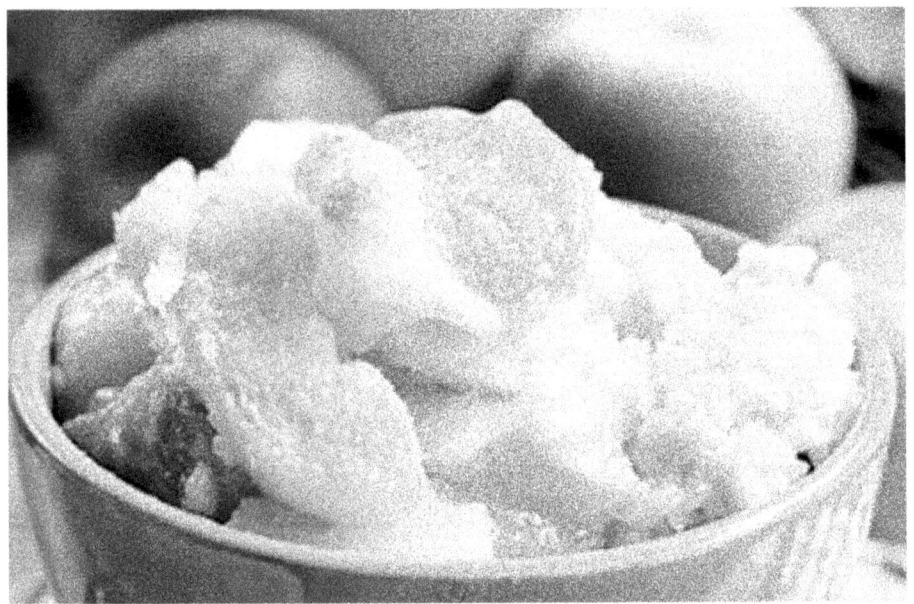

### Ingredients:

- 1 peach, sliced
- 1 tablespoon white whole-wheat flour
- 2 tablespoons instant oats
- 1 tablespoon brown sugar

- A pinch ground cinnamon
- A pinch ground nutmeg
- 1 tablespoon nondairy milk
- 1 tablespoon vanilla vegan yogurt

**Instructions**:

1. Place peaches in a mug and set aside
2. In a small bowl, whisk flour, instant oats, brown sugar, a pinch of ground cinnamon and a pinch of ground nutmeg.
3. Stir in nondairy milk.
4. Pour the oat mixture on top of the peaches and microwave 1–2 minutes, until the oat topping looks a little like oatmeal.
5. Serve hot with your favorite toppings.

**Nutritional Information**: 126 calories per serving, 28.5g carbs, 0.9g fat, 2.7g protein, 2.7g fiber

# Raw Apple Crumble

**Servings**: 4

**Prep Time**: 15 Minutes
**Cook Time**: 0 Minutes

This is a great desert to make because it requires no baking. The flavors come from whole foods and not bad-for-you additives.

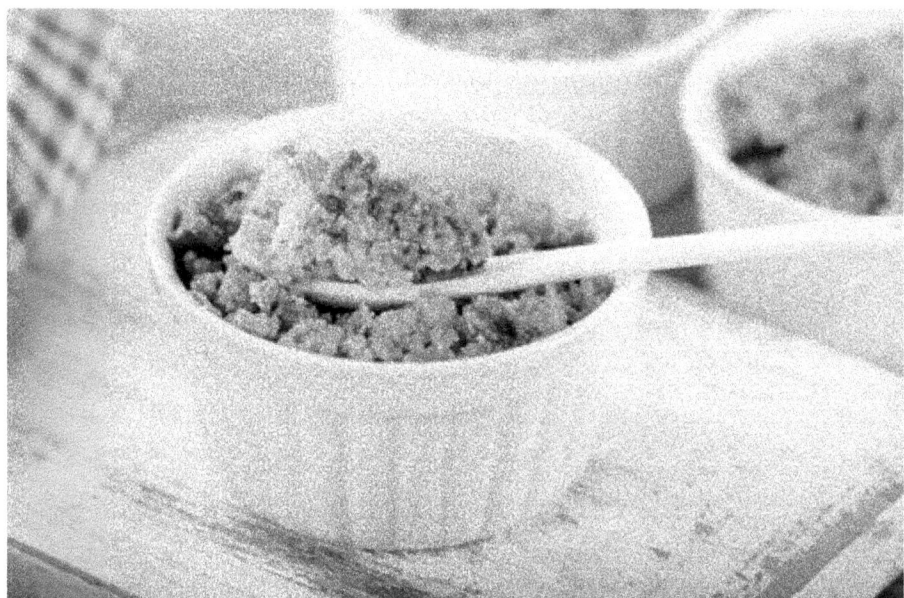

### Ingredients:

- 1 cup walnuts
- 4 pitted dates
- 5 apples, largely diced
- 3 tablespoon lemon juice
- 6 pitted Medjool dates
- ¼ teaspoon cinnamon
- ¼ teaspoon nutmeg

**Instructions**:

1. Starting with the topping, blend the walnuts and 4 dates in a blender or food processor. Transfer this mix into a small bowl.
2. Moving on to the filling, toss 3 apples with 1 tablespoon of lemon juice and set aside.
3. Place the remaining 2 chopped apples into a blender or food processor and blend along with 2 tablespoons of lemon juice, 6 pitted dates, cinnamon and nutmeg.
4. Once blended, pour it onto the apples you set aside and toss.
5. Serve the filling in small dessert dishes and cover with the date-nut topping.

*Tip: Some good suggestions as to what apples to use are Gala or Fiji.*

**Nutritional Information**: 339 calories per serving, 41g carbs, 10g fat, 8g protein, 8g fiber

# Dark Chocolate Brownies

**Servings**: 20

**Prep Time**: 15 Minutes
**Cook Time**: 20 Minutes

Honestly, is there anything better than a nice moist, chocolatey brownie? Didn't think so. These brownies are chewy, rich and fudgey and best of all-vegan!

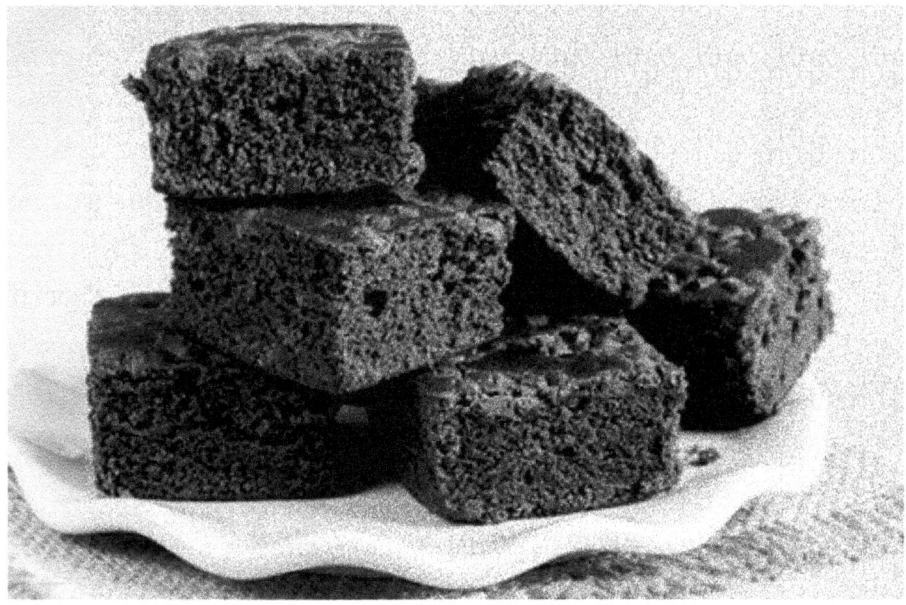

**Ingredients**:

- ¼ cup pureed avocado
- 1 cup white whole-wheat flour
- ½ cup unsweetened cocoa powder
- ¾ cup cane sugar
- 1 teaspoon baking soda
- ½ teaspoon salt
- ¾ cup water

- 1 ½ cups vegan semisweet chocolate chips

**Instructions**:

1. Preheat oven to 350F.
2. In a large mixing bowl, mix together the pureed avocado, flour, cocoa powder, sugar, baking soda, salt and water. Stir all of the ingredients until smooth. Fold in 1 cup of the chocolate chips.
3. Pour into a nonstick baking pan creating an even layer. Sprinkle with an additional ½ cup of chocolate chips on top. Bake for 15-20 minutes.
4. Let cool and serve.

**Nutritional Information**: 30 calories per serving, 5.8g carbs, 0.8g fat, 1.3g protein, 1.5g fiber

# Piña Colada Smoothie

**Servings**: 1

**Prep Time**: 5 Minutes
**Cook Time**: 5 Minutes

This smoothie will have you dreaming of beaches and sunshine. It's smooth and tasty, with none of the bad stuff.

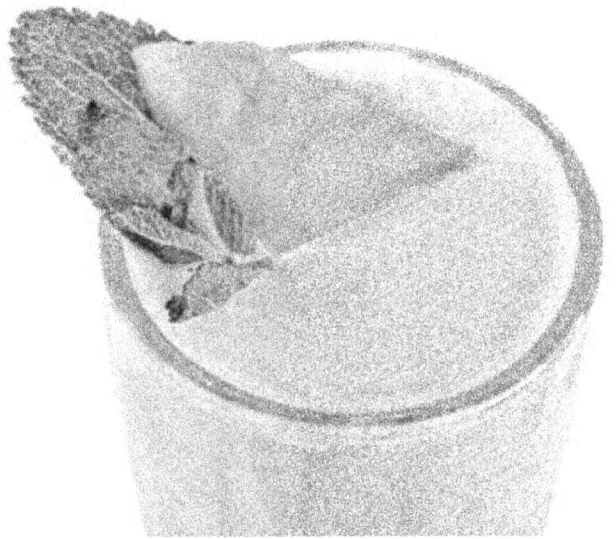

**Ingredients**:

- 1 Frozen Banana
- 1 Cup Pineapple
- 1¼ Cup Rice Milk
- 1 teaspoon Coconut Extract
- ¼ teaspoon Vanilla Extract

**Instructions**:

1. Add all the ingredients into a blender and blend!

*Tip:* When a recipe calls for coconut milk you can use coconut extract added to rice or almond milk.

**Nutritional Information**: 190 calories per serving, 48.8g carbs, 0.6g fat, 2.2g protein, 5.4g fiber

# Chocolate Mousse

**Servings**: 2

**Prep Time**: 5 Minutes
**Cook Time**: 5 Minutes

> This mousse is great for when you are having a chocolate craving. This healthier mousse recipe is rich, creamy and satisfying.

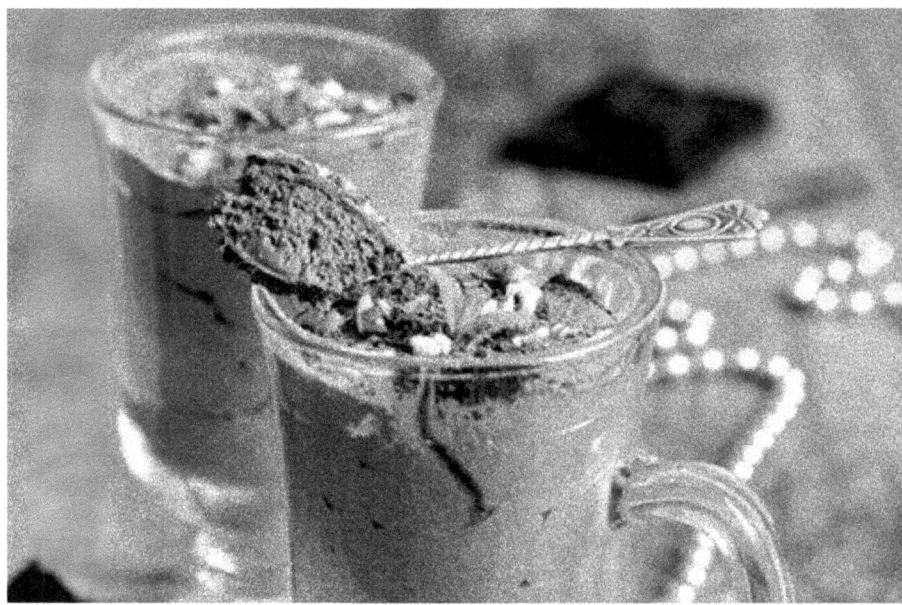

## Ingredients:

- 1 ½ cups rice milk
- 6 tablespoons unsweetened cocoa
- ¼ teaspoon peppermint extract
- vegan chocolate chips

## Instructions:

1. Whisk together all three ingredients until you begin to

see air bubbles appear.
2. Pour into small dessert bowls or ramekins and place into fridge to set, preferably overnight.
3. Once mousse has set, sprinkle on some chocolate chips and serve.

**Nutritional Information**: 129 calories per serving, 27.5g carbs, 3.7g fat, 3.5g protein, 5.4g fiber

# Banana Cream Pie

**Servings**: 6

**Prep Time**: 1 hour 45 Minutes

These banana cream pies may be mini, but they pack a delicious punch. This recipe combines the goodness of bananas, peanut butter and chocolate chips into wonderful small hand held package.

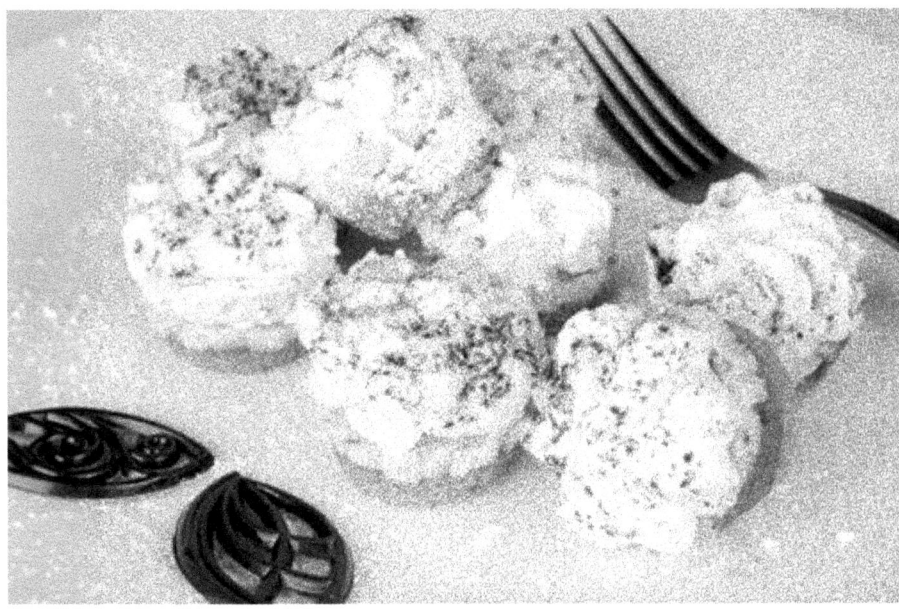

**Ingredients**:

- ½ cup large pitted medjool dates
- ½ cup sunflower butter
- ¼ cup ground flax seed
- ½ cup dry rolled oats
- 2 tablespoons water
- 1 cup cashews
- 1 large ripe banana
- ¼ tablespoon vanilla

- ¼ teaspoon fine sea salt
- 2 tablespoons lemon juice
- 1 tablespoon water

**Instructions**:

1. To begin working on the crust, add dates into a bowl and cover with boiling water. Let soak for 15 minutes then drain.
2. Add the dates, peanut butter, flax seed, rolled oats and 2 tablespoons of water to a food processor or a blender.
3. Pulse the ingredients until they start to clump together.
4. Use a spatula to scrape the mixture into a bowl. Roll the mixture into 6 dough balls.
5. Line a muffin tin with six small sheets of plastic wrap, then place a dough ball in each lined cup.
6. Press down the center of the dough and work it out towards the edges of the cup until it covers the cup in a thin layer.
7. Place the crusts in the refrigerator and move on to work on the filling.
8. Place cashews into a bowl and cover with boiling water. Allow to soak for 30 minutes then drain.
9. Add cashews, banana, vanilla, lemon, salt and water to a cleaned food processer.
10. Blend on high until mixture is creamy.
11. Remove the crust from the refrigerator. Spoon the filling into each crust and refrigerate for at least one hour before serving.
12. Once the pies have set remove them from the tin by pulling up on the plastic wrap. Carefully remove the plastic wrap and serve.

**Nutritional Information**: 205 calories per serving, 18.8g carbs, 12g fat, 5.6g protein, 3.2g fiber

# Apple Strudel

**Servings**: 1

**Prep Time**: 5 Minutes
**Cook Time**: 15 Minutes

This recipe for a traditional Austrian dessert can be made using only 3 ingredients. It's perfect for a quick dessert or to show off some baking skills for some guests.

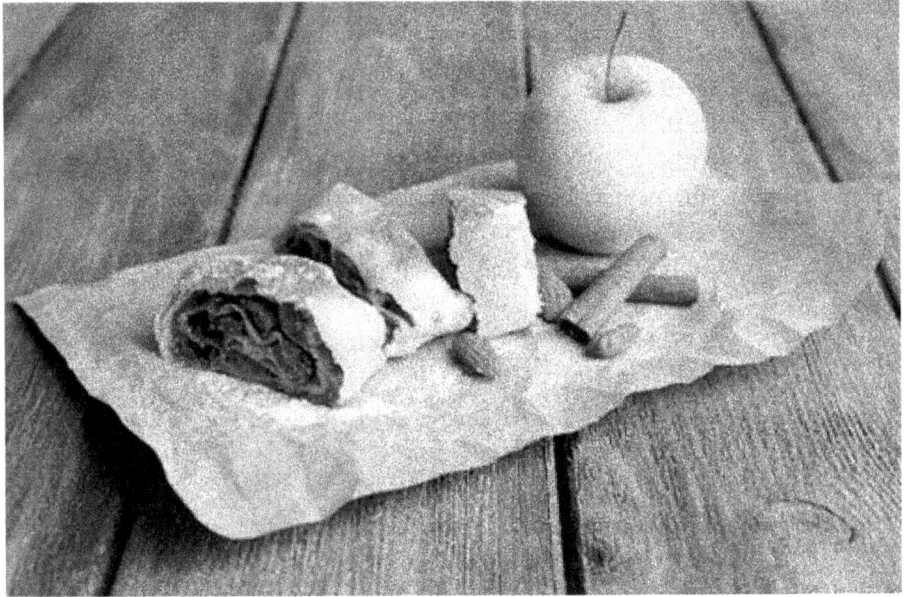

### Ingredients:

- 1 package vegan puff pastry dough
- 2 apples
- ¾ teaspoon cinnamon

### Instructions:

1. Pre-heat oven to 350°F.
2. Remove the pastry dough from the refrigerator and

allow to thaw.
3. Peel the apples and get rid of the seeds.
4. Slice the apples into very thin slices.
5. Add the cinnamon to the apple slices and mix well.
6. Place the apples onto the pastry dough (which should now be on a baking pan) and fold it in then close the edges.
7. Place the apple strudel into the oven and bake for about 15 minutes.
8. Once the strudel is finished baking, serve.

**Nutritional Information**: 194 calories per serving, 51g carbs, 0.7g fat, 1g protein, 9.7g fiber

# NEW – Available Now

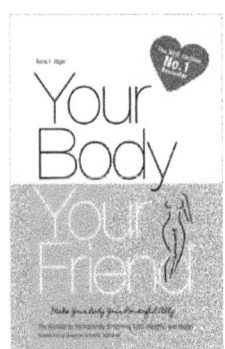

**The NEW German No. 1 Bestseller:
Your Body, Your Friend**

The Answer to Permanently Becoming Slim, Healthy, and Happy
*Based on Scientific Research*

**Fat Storer Goodbye!
Fat Burner Hello.**

In the course of her research, bestselling author and long-time nutritionist Anna I. Jäger discovered a fairly simple, logical solution: We need to stop fighting against the biologically natural processes of the organism that we call our bodies. We need to, instead, join forces with them! A healthy, well nourished body will run more efficiently and lose its extra pounds automatically.

No, these are not false promises; this is biology.

**Your Body Needs Energy to Heal
Your Body Needs Energy to Feel Happy
Your Body Needs Energy to Burn Fat (!)**

As you read through these chapters, you'll learn:

- How to train your body to become a fat burner, not a fat storer
- Why cutting calories is dangerous for your mind and body
- Why low carb diets will make you gain more fat longterm
- How to overcome an eating disorder
- How to lower your set-point (the weight your body tries to maintain)

**Make Your Body Your Powerful Ally**

Get this book so you can learn how you can transform your body and life starting today by becoming best friends with your body and nourishing yourself into a new, slim, healthy, and happy you!

ISBN-13: 978-1508525448
ISBN-10: 1508525447

# Recommendations

**Recommended books on nutrition:**

**T. Colin Campbell, Thomas M. Campbell**
The China Study
The Most Comprehensive Study of Nutrition Ever Conducted And the Startling Implications for Diet, Weight Loss, And Long-term Health

**Dr. John A. McDougall, MD**
The Starch Solution
Eat the foods you love, regain your health, and lose the weight for good

**Dr. Neal Bernard, MD**
Power Foods for the Brain
An Effective 3-Step Plan to Protect Your Mind and Strengthen Your Memory
21-Day Weight Loss Kickstart
Boost Metabolism, Lower Cholesterol, and Dramatically Improve Your Health
Dr. Neal Barnard's Program for Reversing Diabetes
The Scientifically Proven System for Reversing Diabetes without Drugs

**Dr. Caldwell B. Esselstyn Jr.**
Prevent and Reverse Heart Disease
The Revolutionary, Scientifically Proven, Nutrition-Based Cure

# Disclaimer & Legal Information

This book is intended as a reference volume only, not as a medical manual. Nothing written in this book should be viewed as a substitute for competent medical care. The information given here is designed to help you make more informed decisions about your health. It is not intended as a substitute for any treatment that may have been prescribed by your doctor. If you suspect that you have a medical problem, we urge you to seek competent medical help. Also, you should not undertake any changes in diet or exercise patterns without first consulting your physician, especially if you are currently being treated for any risk factor related to heart disease, high blood pressure or adult-onset diabetes. If you follow a low-fat vegan plan strictly for more than 3 years, or if you are pregnant and nursing, then consult your physician in regard to taking a minimum of 5 micrograms of supplemental vitamin B12 daily.

Neither the publisher nor the author disengaged in rendering professional advice or services to the individual reader. Neither the author nor the publisher shall be liable or responsible for any loss or damage allegedly arising from any information or suggestion in this book.

Mention of specific companies, organizations or authorities in this book does not imply endorsement by the publisher, nor does mention of specific companies, organizations, or authorities imply that they endorse the book. Further, the publisher does not have any control over and does not assume any responsibility for author or third-party websites or their content.

No part of this publication may be reproduced or transmitted in any form or by any means, electronic or mechanical, including photocopying, recording, or any other information storage and retrieval system, without the written permission from the copyright owner.

The information in the *7-Day Mealplan Recipes* is true and complete to the best of our knowledge. *7-Day Mealplan Recipes* is intended only as an informative guide for those wanting to know more about food, cooking, health, and environmental issues.

Every effort has been made to ensure the accuracy of the information presented and any claims made. However it is the responsibility of the reader to ensure the suitability of the product and recipe for their particular needs. If you or anyone likely to be consuming food from the *7-Day Mealplan Recipes*, has any food allergies or sensitivities, it is your responsibility to ensure all ingredients are checked before use. The author and publisher make no guarantee as to the availability of products in this book. Many ingredients vary in size and texture and these differences may affect the outcome of some recipes.

In no way is the *7-Day Mealplan Recipes* and those attached to it, intended to replace, countermand, or conflict with the advice given to you by your own doctor or other physician. If you know or suspect that you have a health problem, professional medical or nutritional advice should be sought for any specific issues before embarking on any dietary changes. The ultimate decision concerning care should be made between you and your doctor. We strongly recommend that you follow their advice.

Information in the *7-Day Mealplan Recipes* is general and is offered with no guarantees on the part of the author or the publisher. The author and publisher disclaim all liability in connection with the use of the *7-Day Mealplan Recipes*.

Copyright © A. I. Jäger

All rights reserved. No part of this publication may be reproduced or transmitted in any form or by any means, electronic or mechanical, including photocopying, recording, or any other information storage and retrieval system, without the written permission from the copyright owner except in the case of brief quota-tions or brief quotations embodied in critical articles or reviews.

„Taking the Vegan Challenge;

A Guide to Going Vegan to Lose up to 20 Pounds in 30 Days;
Vegan Diet For Weight Loss incl. Recipes"
by Jäger, A., I.;

Series: Vegan Diet for Beginners

Published by: A.I. Jäger

First Edition January 2015

(Version 2.0)

Image rights: Cover image
© Can Stock Photo Inc. / yadviga
© Brad Pict - Fotolia.com

Updated January 27th 2016

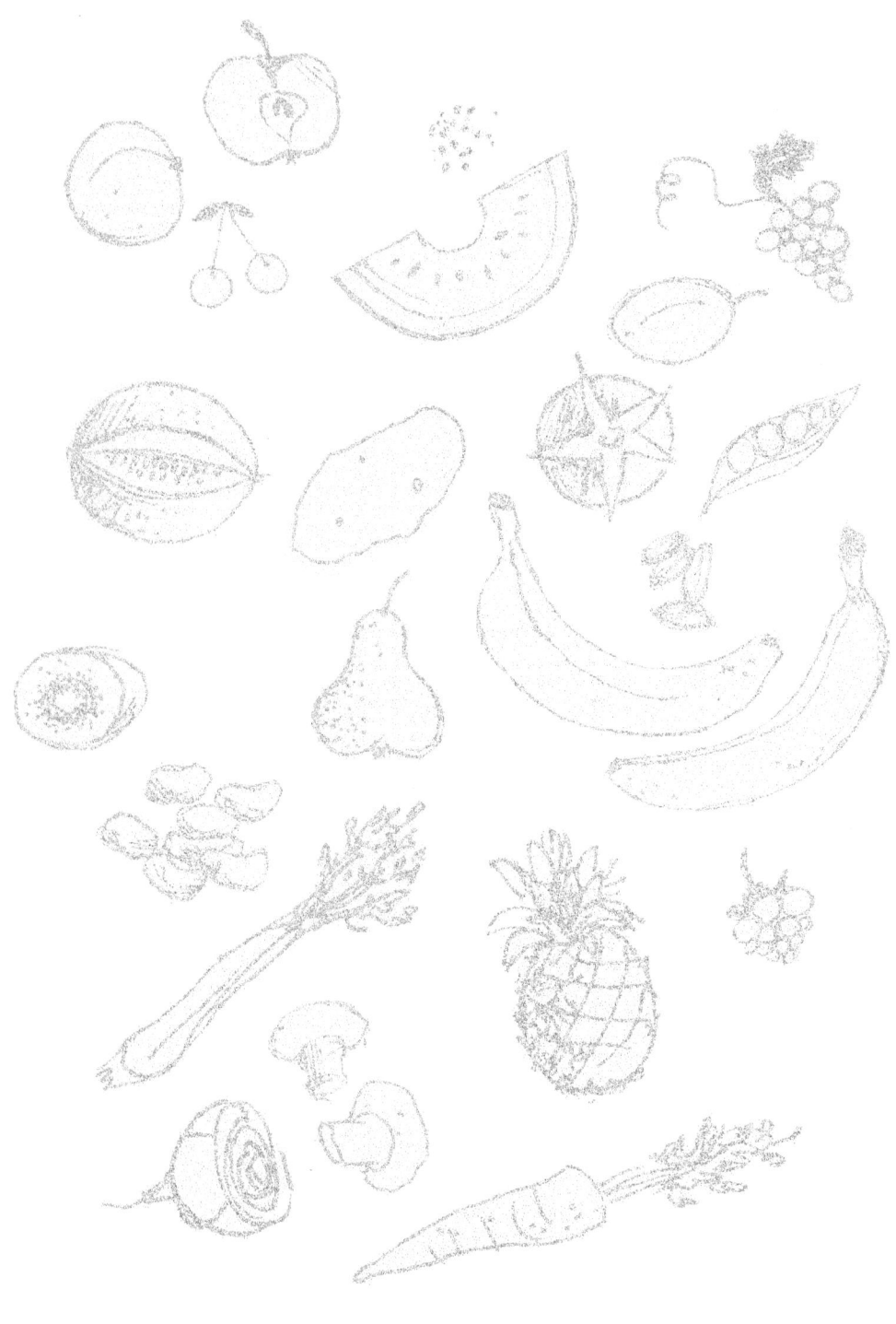

Lightning Source UK Ltd.
Milton Keynes UK
UKHW02f2151270818
327885UK00030B/1367/P